Finding Grace and Balance in the Cycle of Life:

Exploring Integrative Gynecology

Claudia E. Harsh, MD

iUniverse, Inc.
New York   Bloomington

Finding Grace and Balance in the Cycle of Life
Exploring Integrative Gynecology

iUniverse books may be ordered through booksellers or by contacting:

iUniverse
1663 Liberty Drive
Bloomington, IN 47403
www.iuniverse.com
1-800-Authors (1-800-288-4677)

ISBN: 978-1-4502-1584-8 (pbk)
ISBN: 978-1-4502-1583-1 (ebk)
ISBN: 978-1-4502-1582-4 (hbk)

Printed in the United States of America

iUniverse rev. date: 3/30/10

For Mom.
Thanks for your unconditional love, support and encouragement.

Contents

Acknowledgments

Many of the chapters in this book started as a column entitled "Be Well" in the *Cincinnati Women's Magazine*. My thanks to the editor and the publisher for their support and encouragement.

My colleagues at the Alliance Institute for Integrative Medicine in Cincinnati keep me learning and growing in functional and integrative medicine. I am honored and blessed to have the opportunity to work with all of them.

The Integrative Medicine Fellowship at the University of Arizona has exposed me to intelligent, compassionate, committed colleagues and mentors too numerous to count. I offer them my gratitude and honor their contribution to my personal perceptions and reflections.

The blessings of my high priestess sisters keep me grounded and awake as we remember and honor ancient patterns together.

The conscious listening of my husband challenges me to explain, to clarify, and to bask in right hemispheric wonder.

The love of my family and friends underlies it all.

Introduction

The universities do not teach all things, so a doctor must seek out old wives, gypsies, sorcerers, wandering tribes, old robbers, and such outlaws and take lessons from them.

Paracelsus, European physician 1493–1541

Our current health care system has a large array of drugs, laboratory services and imaging technology. When the issue is a broken bone, a heart attack or an acute infection such as pneumonia, the current system is stellar! We train doctors in hospitals that are full of acutely ill people. We learn as interns from residents and attending physicians. We spend time with textbooks and reference articles and then translate that knowledge into helping patients with broken bones, heart attacks and pneumonia. We learn from repetition and practice. We learn the different treatments depending on which bone is broken or what type of bacteria or virus is causing the pneumonia. I spent four years of medical school and a good portion of my residency learning acute care medicine; and as grateful as I am for my Western medical training and experience, I recognize that the majority of my practice is not acute care medicine.

After residency training I moved into a private practice and immediately recognized that the acute care paradigm for health care didn't translate into excellent care for chronic illnesses such as fatigue, chronic pain, weight loss, arthritis, diabetes and uterine fibroids. It is in this framework that Paracelsus' words start to make sense. Where should we find the knowledge and perspectives we need? Perhaps "old wives, gypsies, and sorcerers" represented the ancient traditions of healing in the mind of Paracelsus. This book is a result of over twenty years of exploration and experience in these areas.

My own Western medical training taught me gynecology as it is known and practiced in our culture. I was honored with excellent teachers and mentors throughout my training. Medical school, residency training and postgraduate courses are built on science and learned truth that has gradually shifted and changed into our current understanding of the anatomy and physiology of our bodies. There is a learning curve that we all follow in medicine to reach the medical "standard of care." This standard of care is based on our experiences and the research of the time. I am struck by how the learning curve seems to flatten for many of my colleagues—as if all the questions were answered and there was no need to continue to ask any more questions! Moreover, new ideas and different perspectives cause the "old guard" to become defensive and suspicious. I believe this is not because they want less than optimal care for their patients, but because they're not aware of the new science and its implications and therefore aren't ready to shift their perspective. They're not aware either because they are inundated with paperwork and responsibilities of patient care or because they just haven't looked beyond the narrow perspective of their own subspecialty peer-reviewed journals.

I realize that the standard of care is based on "how it's always been done," and innovation in medical care comes from *interventions* such as prescription drugs and surgical tools.

Marketing these interventions to physicians and the public becomes the focus, rather than exploring and providing a balanced perspective on health. Our peer-reviewed literature often consists of drug trials or instrumentation trials funded by the drug or medical instrument company pushing for acceptance and routine use.

I've seen new gynecological procedures introduced and accepted again and again without looking at what could be done less invasively and more safely to and for women. Most clinical trials that involve taking chemicals *into* our bodies provide no discussion or measurement of our individual differences in metabolizing the same chemicals *out of* our bodies. Our genetic uniquenesses are likely to drive this discussion in ten to fifteen years. For now, these studies lump us together as if we were identical metabolically, physiologically and genetically. The mentors in my field of gynecology are often paid to do the research and present the results; what's more, there are "Committee Opinions" published by our professional organizations that parrot the results and steer the standard of care.

As an example, an ob-gyn (obstetrician-gynecologist) physician wrote a recent article in the magazine *Menopause Management,* which is published by the North American Menopause Society, on the different types of low dose hormone replacement therapy (Warren, 2008). I was amazed to see that she listed as disclosures that she has served as a consultant for Barr Laboratories, Bradley Pharmaceuticals, Warner Chilcott and Novo Nordisk pharmaceuticals. She has also served on speakers' bureaus for Eli Lilly, Merck, Novartis, Nova Nordisk and Wyeth Pharmaceuticals. Furthermore, Nova Nordisk *funded* the preparation of the manuscript through an unrestricted grant. I can't help but believe that her perspective might include an industry bias. And yet this type of review article will be cited and quoted and held up as the standard of care until the next review article supported by the big pharmaceutical companies is published.

Far from a flattened learning curve,. I recognize that we still have much to learn about the intricacies of our bodies. We have unlocked the human genome and are only beginning to understand the weblike interconnectedness that exists between our genetic make-up and how we are designed to respond to our surroundings. As you continue to read, I hope I can share a glimmer of the wonder that I see in the evolving awareness of this field.

I owned a private ob-gyn practice for fourteen years with some wonderful colleagues. Like most ob-gyn physicians, we were pushed to see more clients in a day and to perform more clinical procedures to meet the financial pressures of our business. Western medical practitioners have seen their reimbursements decrease or remain flat in the context of an environment that has seen the rest of our costs continue to rise. Insurance companies did not (and still do not) reimburse for prolonged educational conversations with patients, and I found that some topics were just not suitable for our standard yearly exam in the allotted thirty minutes. (I also knew of colleagues who booked their yearly exams every fifteen minutes or less!) I couldn't fully explore time-intensive topics that came up such as marital stress or pregnancy loss or a child with special needs. In addition it was difficult to have a thorough discussion of nutrition and lifestyle coaching. Through the course of my private practice I felt gradually less fulfilled and less connected to women's health and well-being.

Not only did I realize that areas such as grief counseling for pregnancy loss or lactation counseling were time-rich and reimbursement-poor, I also began to recognize that the traditional Western approaches didn't fully explain or solve my patients' problems. As an example, I started to see a correlation between a woman's social history and her menstrual bleeding. More than once I noticed that the patient who needed a hysterectomy was either in the middle of a divorce or in some sort of family crisis. It took me a while to figure out how to encourage my clients to pay attention to what they saw as "extraneous" issues as part of the treatment for their bleeding issues. My training and readings expanded from our profession's standard texts to others that were taking a more balanced approach to women's health.

Another example where my Western training didn't fully meet my patients' needs was in dealing with premenstrual syndrome or PMS. Our standard recommendations in Western medicine are a nod to nutrition and exercise and then the prescription of either birth control pills or an antidepressant. (Eli Lilly even repackaged their selective serotonin reuptake inhibitor Prozac when it was going off patent into Serafem to capitalize on this new use.) As you'll see in the chapter on PMS, an awareness of the cycles and the hormonal fluctuations within the cycle can be empowering and affirming rather than oppressive and overwhelming.

Like many of my colleagues, I felt pulled apart by responsibilities and expectations. I was balancing a busy practice and night call with my marriage and family. I began to recognize that there is a rhythm and a pattern and an underlying force of balance in our bodies. Our cultural pattern has become a tendency to *push through* our lives rather than to *live in* them! I felt less connected to the wonders of the cycle of life, and each day was another set of challenges rather than an awareness of blessings. I felt I was modeling the antithesis of life-balance and health for my clients; what's more, my marriage was stressed and our son needed me.

After some careful thought and research, I completed acupuncture training at UCLA and then joined the staff at the Alliance Institute for Integrative Medicine in Cincinnati, Ohio. These trail-blazing clinicians and staff have reinforced my professional interests and encouraged me to trust what I've come to know and understand about rhythm and balance in women's health care. I honor and acknowledge my colleagues' willingness to explore this *new medicine* with a thorough grounding in both Eastern and Western philosophies. The inter-mixing of disciplines and practitioners is a fertile ground to explore optimal health and personal growth.

One aspect of medicine that we are exploring at the Alliance Institute is functional medicine. This is a dynamic approach to assessing, preventing and treating complex chronic disease. There is a strong effort now to put scientific reasoning behind the physiologic disruptions that up to this point only had somewhat nonspecific symptoms to describe them. Because Western medicine couldn't measure the symptoms (for example, fatigue or nonspecific pain), the symptom was discounted and described pejoratively as "functional" or "psychosomatic." More information can be obtained at the Institute for Functional Medicine's Web site (www.functionalmedicine.org), and practitioners can reference the recently published *Textbook of Functional Medicine*.

From my experience here at the Alliance Institute, I have crystallized an intention to write this book about integrative gynecology. Now that my practice is more consultative gynecology rather than a traditional ob-gyn practice, I have had more time to assess and consider the current standard of care and explore suggestions for a balanced approach to caring for women throughout their lives.

I have been blessed to have teachers and mentors show up in my life at just the right time, although I didn't always recognize them at the time. One mentor, Lisa Michaels, introduced me to the elemental mysteries and the wheel of the year (www. naturalrhythms.org). By right alignment of earth, water, air and fire, I have been honored to witness the dance of spirit in my life. What's more, I see the intricacies of women's health and balance through wider and more inclusive eyes. The simplistic term of mind-body medicine comes into focus as we acknowledge earth (physical realm), water (emotional realm), air (mental realm) and fire (action realm).

The seasons pass from winter to spring to summer to autumn to winter again. There is no time of complete stillness—as long as we are alive, there is always a growth and movement and evolution over time. The earth rotates on its axis, and we see the stars change in relationship to where we are in this given moment in time. The moon waxes and wanes and waxes again. We start our development as eggs inside our mother's ovaries inside our grandmother's womb. We are pushed into a unique dance of existence that we can only begin to appreciate as the years unfold.

The Psalmist says in Psalm 139, verses 13 and 14 (NIV): *For you created my inmost being; you knit me together in my mother's womb. I praise you because I am fearfully and wonderfully made; your works are wonderful, I know that full well.*

We are genetically unique and yet can turn on and off our genetic predispositions with our nutrition and stresses and exposure through stages of physical, emotional and spiritual changes.

We are babies, then children, then adolescents, then adults and then leave this life for who knows what and where? Amid these changes and cycles I've been blessed to come into the awareness of how the cycles of our lives are clearly affected by the patterns and rhythms of our world.

Let's explore women's health in the awareness of this grace and balance together. The field of integrative gynecology combines the science and traditions of obstetrics and gynecology along with the ancient teachings of Chinese medicine, acupuncture and other alternative teachings. I'll start the discussion with an exploration of nutrition and lifestyle choices and then explore the different phases of a woman's life in the following chapters. I honor your interest and thank you for joining me on the journey.

1

Lifestyle Choices and Habits

Everyone should be his own physician. We ought to assist and not force nature. Eat with moderation and with what agrees with your constitution. Nothing is good for the body but what we can digest. What medicine can produce digestion? Exercise. What will recruit strength? Sleep. What will alleviate incurable ills? Patience.

Voltaire (1694–1778)

This chapter contains the basics for women's health and wellness. If you browse through no other part of the book, take this one to heart. It has become clear that nutrition, stress management and exercise are the keys to emotional, mental, physical and spiritual health. I fully believe that the majority of gynecological disorders are imbalances that can be prevented or corrected with attention to these areas.

We are reluctant to believe this as a culture. There has been a push for "evidence-based medicine" that is often more aptly described as "intervention-based medicine." A study from Australia, for example, showed that the "lap band" (laparoscopic adjustable gastric banding—a form of bariatric or weight loss surgery) was a "better" treatment for patients with type 2 diabetes than expectant and routine management (Dixon, 2008). The thirty control patients were treated as any typical patient in the United States is treated; they were told to walk 10,000 steps a day and participate in a regular structured exercise program. There was a nod to nutrition guidelines but no discussion of stress management or life pacing or counseling. The common denominator for remission in both groups was successful weight loss.

I wasn't surprised to learn that 73 percent of the patients who had the surgery achieved remission of their diabetes within two years, versus 13 percent of the control group. The surgical group had a higher percentage of people with weight loss, so they had a higher percentage of people with diabetes remission. Six of the thirty patients in the surgical group had some type of surgical complication. One band had to be surgically removed two weeks after it was placed.

Besides the concern that there was no "active management" control group where health coaching, stress management and aggressive nutrition counseling was in place, I'm left wondering why we are drawn to forces outside ourselves for solutions to our health problems. What causes us to overeat foods that increase our weight and our diabetes risk? Why isn't there more public outcry when giant food processing companies subvert health and nutrition with marketing and glitz that cover up empty calories and dangerous fats? There's no doubt we're addicted to sugar as a culture; I'm hopeful we can explore this addiction and awaken to its dangers. It's all brain chemistry—pleasure chemicals are triggered and exploited. We get the "why"—now let's problem-solve for solutions.

Resolving to Change

As the New Year comes each year it brings with it a sense of renewal and optimism. It's natural to look at the stretch of days unfolding before us and dream. What do we want to bring into our lives? What do we want to remove? Setting intentions is the best way to transform our lives. Yet, it is depressing to read that over 60 percent of New Year's resolutions are broken within the first half of the year. Whether it's addictions to cigarettes, or broken promises to eat healthy or exercise, we haven't quite found the strategies as a culture to control our urges and impulses. (I'm frequently asked for that special acupuncture needle that will control sugar cravings! Guess what? It's more complicated than that.)

Three psychologists, James Prochaska, John Norcross and Carlo DiClemente, studied "self-changers" or people who had successfully stopped smoking or lost weight or started an exercise program and recognized that all successful behavior changers pass through six stages of change that are distinct and measurable. Their book *Changing for Good* (Prochaska, 1994) should be a guide for anyone interested in setting intentions or resolutions. The six stages of change are:
- precontemplation
- contemplation
- preparation
- action
- maintenance

- termination

The authors describe the process of change as a spiral—not a linear step-by-step progression. We'll review the stages below and discuss how to apply them in your own life to habits you'd like to change.

- Precontemplation: People who are in the precontemplation stage of change are usually not making New Year's resolutions. They don't see their health habits as problems, and if they show up in therapy or at an exercise class, for example, it's usually because they were pushed to go by a spouse or friend. As you can imagine, if you or someone you know are in the precontemplation stage, you're not going to change your behavior successfully without insight and education. Sometimes the impetus to change is a health scare. A patient, Betty (not her real name), has smoked for over thirty years. She's quit smoking a few times for six months or so but always picks up the habit again in response to the stress in her life. She is intelligent and insightful and knows intellectually that smoking is unhealthy. Her hands and ankles are swollen and she's been short of breath. She has stopped smoking as of this week after she developed dizzy spells and fell in her house. In Betty's case, she was moved out of precontemplation by a health scare. She knew intuitively how to stop smoking and immediately and successfully quit. I'm hopeful she'll continue on the path to becoming a nonsmoker and hope to be one of her cheerleaders as she changes this habit.

- Contemplation: Contemplators are at the stage of change where they are aware that they have a problem and may have a degree of frustration with feeling stuck. People at this stage are not quite ready to change; perhaps if they read just one more book or just one more Web site they will find that there's a dream therapy that will curb the urge to smoke or a new supplement that will burn fat. (Marketing people love contemplators. They are most likely to buy their product but will not necessarily put in the time and energy to actually change their behaviors.) Contemplators are essentially stuck in the interminable research phase of understanding their problem and aren't stepping forward yet with an action plan.

- Preparation: On the other hand, if you're in the preparation stage, you've chosen an action plan and have set a time frame within the next month to begin. You're more likely to be successful with your New Year's resolutions if you couple the resolution with a strategy for success. (For example, if weight loss is your goal, clear out all those empty-calorie foods from your house and make sure those cookbooks with fast and easy organic vegetable and whole grain foods are read and marked with bookmarks! Have your shopping list made up and ready. Enlist the support of your family or roommates.) My patient Darine (not her real name) has thought about instituting an exercise program. She joined a gym a few years ago but after about six months didn't attend regularly and got frustrated every time the monthly charge came in. Her strategy this year is to enlist a neighbor who has a similar schedule. They have set up exercise dates and clear concrete goals together. So far, her buddy system is working well and she is pleased with her energy level and stamina.

- Action: In the same way, the action stage is a result of planning and effort, and it is when our behavior is outwardly changing. This stage works hand in hand with the maintenance stage because slipping into old habits will happen unless we're aware of how stresses and pressure in our lives pull us back to old habits. Alcoholics in twelve-step programs such as Alcoholics Anonymous use the awareness of a daily choice and recognize that even one drink is too much *ever*. On the other hand, many of us know someone like Betty who has quit smoking and started again. Changing behaviors is a lifetime daily choice.

- Maintenance: Behavior change is a daily choice combined with strategies that individually apply to who we are and what we need to be successful. Betty knows what some of her triggers are for smoking. She knows that if she sits down in the morning to read the paper she will want a cigarette. She has changed her morning routine as part of her smoking strategy. Darine knows that her exercise program slips when she becomes busy or stressed. Both women recognize their habits require constant attention and vigilance. Until the chosen habit is ingrained and automatic they stay in the maintenance phase of change.

- Termination: No life changing habit is easy. On the other hand, I know several people who are ex-smokers or who have maintained weight loss or exercise programs. The termination phase of the psychology of change is only noticed in retrospect. More than likely, most successful changers remain vigilant and committed to their choices.

Rather than looking out at the horizon, I encourage people in the action stage of change to make weekly goals and then assess the goals at the end of the week and either celebrate or forgive prior to setting the next week's goals. This deceptively simple strategy keeps the intention or the goal at the forefront of our awareness and makes it easier to avoid relapse. We are so prone to self-judgment; if we recognize this at the outset, we will be more able to acknowledge the power of choice in our lives. Changing behaviors that we've had for years is not easy. There's a reason we fell into the behavior in the first place (it feels good, it tastes good, etc.). But that doesn't mean we can't change the behavior with intention and commitment.

Nutrition and Supplements

Are you confused about what to eat for optimal health? Just check out the nutrition section of your local bookstore and look around in confusion. Grapefruit? Blood type? Paleolithic? The variety and level of complexity is mind-boggling. The argument about macronutrients (carbohydrates, fat and protein) has captured our attention in the last decade. Two approaches to nutrition championed by Dean Ornish, MD, (low low fat) and Robert Atkins, MD, (low low carbohydrates) are examples.

Is there a perfect meal and supplement plan for each person on the planet? The science of nutragenomics is exploring this; I expect we'll have better answers within the next five to ten years. At least for now we know that the work of many researchers including Walter Willett, MD, DrPH, of the Harvard School of Public Health is a good starting point. It's clear to me that the modified Mediterranean diet is currently the best approach for all of us for now. The Mediterranean diet uses daily exercise as its base and then recommends whole grains, vegetables, fruit and lean protein (in that order). An excellent resource for information on nutrition is www.oldwayspt.org. In addition to reviewing the Mediterranean diet, this Web site explores traditional cultures and their healthy diets including groups such as vegetarians, Asians, Latin Americans and even modifications for children.

I tell my patients to avoid "white food"—white sugar, white rice, white flour and white pasta. All are associated with increased inflammation in our bodies. I suggest they avoid the middle portion of the grocery store—the canned and processed foods with long shelf lives live there! In order to have a long shelf life, these foods are more likely to have preservatives and additives. Stay on the outside circuit for the fruits, vegetables, lean protein and other healthier choices. I encourage my patients to slow down and relax while they're chewing and to use small plates whenever possible.

Our government has stepped in with opinions through the U.S. Department of Agriculture (USDA). The government's food guide pyramid makes recommendations on the types and amounts of food to be eaten every day. It was updated in 2005 to include not only variety, proportionality and moderation in selecting foods, but also regular physical activity. There is a stick figure climbing stairs on the side of the pyramid to illustrate the point.

In addition to the general recommendations, the USDA has also made specific recommendations for micronutrients (vitamins and minerals) for specific groups of people:

- People over age 50. Consume 25 mcg of vitamin B12 in its crystalline form (i.e., fortified foods or supplements).
- Women of childbearing age who may become pregnant. Eat foods high in heme-iron and/or consume iron-rich plant foods or iron-fortified foods with an enhancer of iron absorption, such as vitamin C–rich foods.
- Women of childbearing age who may become pregnant and those in the first trimester of pregnancy. Consume adequate synthetic folic acid daily (from fortified foods or supplements) in addition to food forms of folate from a varied diet.
- Older adults, people with dark skin, and people exposed to insufficient ultraviolet band radiation (i.e., sunlight). Consume extra vitamin D from vitamin D–fortified foods and/or supplements. (We will explore vitamin D more thoroughly in a later chapter.)

Most of my clients are confused about their supplement regimen. I have seen "vitamin habits" run the gamut from never or rarely taking vitamins to taking upwards of twenty or thirty vitamins and supplements a day. I have mapped out spreadsheets with patients so they can see what their vitamin regimen looks like.

Outcomes from an NIH State of the Science Conference in 2006 stated that Americans spend about $23 billion on vitamins and supplements. As a culture we're bombarded with marketing promises and supplement company research that can provide conflicting and confusing suggestions. More than half of the adults in this country take supplements with the expectation that they will feel better, have greater energy, improved health and less chronic disease because of them. Most of us in the healing professions have had little or no training in nutritional supplements and our knowledge has to be self-taught. Ideally our education comes from sources *other* than the companies that have a vested interest in our prescribing patterns.

Most vitamins are isolated from plants; in fact, there is a lot of data to support the many benefits of a diet that is high in vegetables and fruits. The problem is that commercially grown vegetables have been shown to have lower and lower levels of minerals and vitamins. A Rutgers study in the 1990s compared commercially grown produce to organic produce and noted a marked difference in nutritional value (Smith, 1993). The products themselves have been bred to look nice in the store and have a long shelf life; nutritional concerns are often secondary. So the need for supplemental nutrition in the form of capsules and tablets is probably here to stay.

The term *vitamine* was coined in 1912 by a Polish biochemist Casimir Funk from the Latin *vita* meaning life and *amine* because the vitamin that he isolated, B1 or thiamine, was an amine—a chemical derivative of ammonia. He isolated the vitamin from the husks of rice. He followed in the footsteps of Dr. William Fletcher who noted that 25 percent of asylum inmates in Kuala Lumpur who were fed "polished" rice with the husk removed developed beriberi while only 2 percent of the inmates who were fed "unpolished" rice developed the disease. Similar research in this era resulted in the discovery of ascorbic acid or vitamin C in the prevention of scurvy and other deficiency diseases such as pellagra (niacin or vitamin B3) and rickets (vitamin D).

By definition then, a vitamin is an organic compound found in food that results in a deficiency disease if it is removed from the diet. Large-scale fortification of the food supply here in the

United States started in 1924 with the addition of iodine to salt to prevent goiter, followed by the addition of vitamin D to milk in 1933 to prevent rickets and the addition of thiamin, riboflavin, niacin and iron to flour in 1941. It is rare to see overt deficiency diseases here in our country.

What we are exploring now is the science of optimal nutrition. In other words, how can we measure optimal nutrition at a cellular level? What are our individual genetic needs? How often should levels be assessed? And so on. As in any area of new science there is a healthy debate; some believe all nutrition should be food-based alone and others are proponents of multiple supplements. My personal opinion is that nutrition should be an important focus for health, but that ultimately supplemental vitamins, minerals and other "nutraceuticals" (nutritional pharmaceuticals) should be incorporated for optimal health and wellness if the diet is less than optimal.

The FDA lists nine water-soluble (dissolve in water) vitamins: thiamin (B1), riboflavin (B2), niacin (B3), biotin, folic acid, pantothenic acid (B5), pyridoxine (B6), cobalamin (B12) and vitamin C. There are four fat-soluble (don't dissolve in water) vitamins: vitamins A, D, E and K. Don't get confused by the numbering system of B vitamins. Just know that as medical science advanced, some chemicals that were identified as vitamins lost their vitamin status as more information was discovered.

The government has set the Recommended Dietary Allowances (RDA) for vitamins through the Food and Drug Administration and has defined the RDA as the amount of the nutrient that is sufficient to meet the nutrient requirements of nearly all (9 to 98 percent) of healthy individuals in a particular life stage and gender group. The Institute of Medicine has modified the term to Estimated Average Requirement (EAR), which is the amount of the nutrient that meets the requirements of half of the healthy individuals in a particular life stage or gender group. The Tolerable Upper Intake Level (UL) is the highest average nutrient intake that is likely to pose no risk. As more and more people take supplements, it's clear that there needs to be better science to guide them.

Not only do we *not* know the UL in the case of most vitamins, we don't have good randomized controlled trials of vitamin dosing on a general population. For example, how do we have a placebo control when we're studying vitamins in the general population? Most people receiving the placebo are still eating food that has variable amounts of assorted vitamins in it. Moreover, their gastrointestinal tracts vary in efficiency for absorbing and excreting the vitamins. What are the individual genetic differences in storing the vitamin in question? It's no wonder that the data on the value of taking vitamins are confusing and inconclusive to date.

The other confounding problem is that supplement and vitamin quality is not the same from company to company. Despite their claims, the ingredients listed on the label are not always found in the pills. A recent review by a private laboratory (www.consumerlab.com) found that only ten of twenty-one multivitamins that were tested passed quality standards. The other vitamins dissolved poorly, had toxic levels of lead or other contaminants, or contained more or less than the level of a specific vitamin stated on the label.

Quality Standards for Vitamins and Nutraceuticals

We have certain expectations as vitamin consumers, don't we? We expect that the vitamin or supplement bottle that we purchase is full of pills that match the description on the label of the bottle. We also expect that each pill in the bottle will have no dangerous toxins such as lead or cadmium or mercury. We expect the pill was manufactured in a factory that was free of bacteria, fungi or viruses. In short, we expect consistent quality. One thing I can assure you, supplement quality can't be guaranteed by price. So if it costs more, it doesn't mean it's better made or safer. Glitzy marketing on TV, slick advertising in health food stores or beautiful web pages on the Internet also don't guarantee product quality. So how do you know what supplements to buy? And who can give you reliable advice? I'm bemused when a client is more apt to listen to a clerk in a health food store or the sister of a next-door neighbor who is part of a pyramid marketing company instead of me, but I understand it. Most physicians weren't taught much nutrition in medical school—and most are leery of things they don't know.

So let's talk about vitamins and supplements. Let's review what the government standards are for supplement quality and learn how to choose brands of supplements.

Congress passed the Dietary Supplement Health and Education Act (DSHEA) in 1994, in order to define the FDA's authority to regulate dietary supplements. DSHEA states that nutritional supplements and vitamins should be regulated as foods, meaning that they are assumed to be safe. (Contrast this with prescription drugs, which must undergo clinical trials for safety and efficacy before they're sold to the public.) One thing that DSHEA did for vitamin manufacturers was to improve the growth of the industry. There was a 20 percent increase per year in supplement companies in the years following the passage of the law. Although the boom in growth is currently smaller, most analysts still estimate a healthy 2 to 4 percent growth in the next few years despite our gloomy economic environment.

The FDA outlined Current Good Manufacturing Practices (cGMPs) in June 2007. Manufacturers have been given until 2010 to implement the guidelines. (The timing of cGMP phase-in is determined by the size of the manufacturer.) The cGMP guidelines require that nutraceutical (nutritional pharmaceuticals) companies must test their products and confirm that their labeling is reflective of the bottles' content. Sounds ideal, doesn't it? Unfortunately I (and many of my colleagues) see some major loopholes in the policy including (1) enforcement, (2) a lack of specific analysis methods and (3) the exemption of suppliers of raw materials.

An excellent review of these concerns is outlined by Rick Liva, ND, RPh, in the journal *Integrative Medicine* (Liva, 2007). He notes that the FDA is responsible for inspecting about 80 percent of the U.S. food supply (the USDA is responsible for the other 20 percent such as meat, poultry and dairy). In reality, the FDA has historically inspected only about 1.7 percent of the 80 percent. This number is probably lower now because of cutbacks in government spending. But the real concern is in the area of the raw materials. Dr. Liva notes that in his experience anywhere from 30 to 50 percent of the raw materials that he tests have quality issues. There are so many examples of this—from black cohosh products that don't have the active ingredient in the finished product, to mercury contamination in fish oil pills to too much vitamin A in a multivitamin.

My suggestion is to educate yourself about the company whose product you choose to buy. You can also subscribe to private labs that measure over-the-counter supplement quality and publish monthly reports such as Consumerlab (www.consumerlab.com). It is one of several similar tools to use and apply to your health choices.

There is no doubt in my mind that optimizing our nutrition with healthy organic whole food nutrition is the optimal path to health. I believe that optimizing the levels of vitamins and supplements can enhance the *very essence* of our life force energy. We can measure blood levels of some vitamins such as vitamin D. There are also ways of measuring the intracellular "functional" levels of vitamins and minerals using both urine and blood specimens. We have found that these analyses can help a wide range of symptoms including fatigue, allergies, muscle pain and infertility. Our vitamins and nutritional supplements can help us correct deficiencies in soil depletion and food quality and optimize our body's response to our genetic tendencies. I recognize that the science of optimal nutrition is one that is still growing and changing. We're zeroing in on strategies that make a difference in immune system function, digestive tract function and overall quality of life. There is much more to learn.

You get a "D" in Health

There is an increasing concern that most people around the world have low levels of vitamin D. One recent example is an article by Dr. Lisa Bodnar at the University of Pittsburgh Graduate School of Public Health who studied vitamin D levels in laboring women and their infants (Bodnar, 2007). She states:

"In our study, more than 80 percent of African-American women and nearly half of white women tested at delivery had levels of vitamin D that were too low, even though more than 90 percent of them used prenatal vitamins during pregnancy. The numbers also were striking for their newborns—92.4 percent of African-American babies and 66.1 percent of white infants were found to have insufficient vitamin D at birth."

The standard recommendation by dermatologists and other skin experts is to avoid sunlight and to apply sunscreen liberally and frequently. Like most health issues, however, it just *isn't* a black and white (light and dark? sun and shade?) issue. More and more data are coming out about the benefits of having an adequate vitamin D level. We know that vitamin D helps us absorb calcium and phosphate in our gastrointestinal tract. We know that vitamin D suppresses parathyroid hormone (PTH) and acts on cells known as osteoblasts in our bones to stimulate bone formation and reduce bone loss. Data now suggest that adequate vitamin D may help curb the development and progression of *seventeen* types of cancer including breast, prostate and colon. Vitamin D also plays a role in heart disease, stroke, hypertension, diabetes, chronic pain, muscle weakness, and periodontal disease in addition to autoimmune diseases such as rheumatoid arthritis. Also under study is a suspected but unproven role in the immune response in both multiple sclerosis and HIV/AIDS.

Let's understand how we take in vitamin D and its relationship to sunlight. The formation of vitamin D in our bodies starts at the level of our skin. The two outer layers of our skin, our epidermal and dermal cells, absorb ultraviolet B (UVB) radiation from the sun and convert it to previtamin D3, which is rapidly converted to vitamin D3 or cholecalciferol. The amount of vitamin D3 formed in our skin depends on several factors including how long we're exposed to the sun, the time of day, the latitude, the use of sunscreen, the amount of melanin in our skin and our age. We know that we absorb less UVB as we get older. We also know that higher amounts of melanin in African Americans and Hispanics can block UVB absorption and can cause vitamin D deficiency.

We can also get vitamin D from our nutrition, especially from cold-water fatty fish such as tuna, salmon, herring or mackerel. Lesser amounts of vitamin D can be consumed in fortified milk and milk products, fortified juices and rice or soy beverages. Most multivitamins have 400 IU of vitamin D3. The general rule of thumb is to take in 400 to 1000 IU of vitamin D daily. You can easily absorb this amount in fifteen minutes of noonday sun in the summertime on your bare skin. It's harder to get this much from your nutrition.

Your vitamin bottle label may say that it has "vitamin D2" or "ergocalciferol" in it. Vitamin D2 is derived from plants and has been used for over fifty years for symptomatic vitamin D deficiency. Many researchers claim that vitamin D3 should be used instead of vitamin D2. At this point, the data point to preferring vitamin D3, but there are strongly worded discussions still at play in the medical literature.

Once we've made vitamin D3 in our skin, it is rapidly metabolized in the liver to form 25-hydroxy vitamin D3 (25-OH D3), which is the main form of circulating vitamin D in our bodies. Your 25-OH D3 level should be measured by your caregiver to confirm your vitamin D status. Our local lab lists the normal range as 20 to 100 ng/ml. We strongly recommend that you get your 25-OH D3 level to the 50 to 70 ng/ml range. (We'll push the levels higher for clients with severe autoimmune diseases, but we'll screen levels regularly to insure they are not over treated.)

Vitamin D is a fat-soluble vitamin that can build to toxic levels if it isn't monitored closely. On the other hand, if levels are too low, it can take several months to build up fat stores of the vitamin. Obese patients need higher doses of vitamin D for longer periods of time. In addition, clients with a genetic uniqueness of their vitamin D receptor known as a single nucleotide polymorphism, SNP or "snip," are less able to store the vitamin and will need a higher dose.

I'm suggesting that all of my patients get a baseline screening 25-OH D3 level if they have any chronic health problems. This includes chronic pain conditions, autoimmune problems, or a strong family history of cancer or diabetes. I supplement and then recheck the level until the optimal dosing of vitamin D3 is determined. For some people the best dose is 400 IU daily, for some it is 2000 IU daily. Some people need 50,000 IU weekly for three months to build up their stores and then 1000 to 2000 IU daily. I also discuss seasonal variations in dosing, such as a lower dose in the summer time for my clients who are active outdoors. I disagree with "one dose fits all" and suggest that following vitamin D levels is the ideal way to know how much of this important vitamin to take.

Strategies to Combat Free Radicals

Did you think this integrative medicine book had morphed somehow into current events and politics? The news is often filled with stories about radicals, war, aggression and posturing that leave me wondering why more of us "moderates" aren't standing up and speaking out for peace and balance and mediation. But that's not the kind of radicals I'm talking about. I'm talking about the kind of radicals that are waging war inside you and causing cell damage leading to inflammation. This kind of inflammation causes a variety of problems including heart disease, Alzheimer's and cancer. By virtue of breaking down food or taking some medicines or living in our (frequently toxic) environment, we're exposed to free radicals. A free radical is a chemical compound that is unstable—and it's looking for ways to become stable or inert. Understanding all of this instability starts with the concept of chemical bonds. Let's look deep within the cells for a moment and review the very building blocks of life.

The cells in your body are made up of molecules, which are made up of combinations of atoms. Each atom is made up of a nucleus that contains protons and neutrons and rings of electrons that "orbit" the nucleus and react with other atoms by forming chemical bonds. The number of protons within the nucleus determines the number of electrons in the orbits. (Each chemical has a different number of protons—for instance, hydrogen has one, carbon has six, oxygen has eight.) The electrons fill "shells" of orbits; when the outer orbit of electrons is full, the compound is considered stable or inert. In order to fill its outer orbit, atoms exchange electrons and form chemical bonds with other atoms.

Free radicals, then, are formed when a molecule breaks apart either by metabolism or because its chemical bonds are weak. The molecules are unstable with openings in its outer electron orbits causing them to react quickly with nearby molecules to "steal" electrons and cause these "donor" molecules to change, sometimes even making more free radicals. The process can cascade and ultimately disrupt normal cell function. Not all free radicals are bad. Your immune system uses this process to disrupt viruses and other invaders.

Free radicals become a problem when they form in such large numbers that they overwhelm the normal cell's ability to "police"

Claudia E. Harsh, MD

them or neutralize them and cause them to become inert. We've know for a long time that a group of chemicals called antioxidants can neutralize the free radicals by donating an electron. The antioxidants don't become free radicals themselves because they are stable in either their original form or after they've released an electron. Examples of antioxidants include vitamin E, vitamin C, beta-carotene (the water-soluble precursor for vitamin A), and the mineral selenium.

Antioxidants are found in colorful fruits and vegetables. Two recent studies measured different foods and the amount of antioxidants in them. Pomegranates, berries, walnuts, sunflower seeds, ginger, red beets, chili peppers, kale, red cabbage, bell peppers, parsley, artichokes, currants, fava beans, dried apricots and prunes were all high on the antioxidant list in a Norwegian study (Halvorsen, 2002). An Italian study compared three different strategies for measuring antioxidant content, and their top foods were spinach, artichokes, peppers and berries (Pellegrini, 2003). The beverages with the highest antioxidant content were coffee followed by citrus juices. The oils with the highest antioxidant content were soybean and extra virgin olive oil.

The bottom line recommendation of four to five servings of (preferably organic) fruits and vegetables a day still seems to be your best bet for optimal antioxidant function.

Many people take vitamin supplements that contain antioxidants such as vitamin C, vitamin E, selenium and beta-carotene. I've frequently run into patients who think that "if a little is good then a lot is better." Unfortunately, when it comes to antioxidants in supplement form, I have to express some caution. The National Cancer Institute summarizes five studies on its Web site that looked at the use of antioxidants and cancer prevention. Beta-carotene was found to increase lung cancer rates in two studies but had no effect on cancer rates in another. On the other hand, a Chinese study in people with an increased risk of stomach cancer showed a positive effect (less cancer) with extra vitamin E, selenium and beta-carotene (You, 2005). Two important points come to mind: (1) until we understand our genetic uniquenesses and why some of us are prone to develop cancer, we can't make a blanket "one size fits all" recommendation about antioxidant doses. We can, however, measure antioxidant levels in our blood and personalize recommendations. And finally (2) I can't stress enough that until quality control in the nutraceutical industry is standardized and reliable, it is the consumer's responsibility to ask about it again and again.

Here's hoping for a peaceful solution to your inner free radicals.

Cruciferous Vegetables: What, Why and How Much?

I do not like broccoli. And I haven't liked it since I was a little kid and my mother made me eat it. And I'm President of the United States and I'm not going to eat any more broccoli.

George H.W. Bush, March 1990

The forty-first President of the United States caused uproar among broccoli growers with this statement at a press conference two decades ago. Pundits and talk-show hosts found the comment amusing. Broccoli growers around the nation sent truckloads of the vegetable to the White House in response. (Perhaps they thought they could change his mind?) At any rate, we know more now about broccoli than we did in 1990. We know now that the whole class of vegetables that includes broccoli called cruciferous or brassica vegetables are chock full of nutrients and vitamins. And we're beginning to understand their importance in the context of our overall nutrition and health.

In this section we're going to learn why we should all eat our vegetables and how much we should eat daily or weekly. (And for those of you out there who don't want to read about vegetables, "you have to have at least three small bites." That was my parents' rule!)

To start with, what are cruciferous vegetables? They are a group of vegetables that are in the same botanical family known as Cruciferae or Brassicaceae. The family includes broccoli, Brussels sprouts, cabbage, cauliflower, collard greens, kale, kohlrabi, mustard, rutabaga, turnips, bok choy and Chinese cabbage. Arugula, horseradish, radish, wasabi and watercress are also cruciferous vegetables. As a family, the leaves of the plants come out at right angles to one another, which explains the reason for the "cruciform" or cross-forming name of the plant group.

The cruciferous family of vegetables has a widely different flavor from one type to another; however, a unifying theme is a pungent (some say bitter) flavor with chewing. This flavor is caused by a group of chemicals called glucosinolates, which are sulfur-containing chemicals. When chewed, these glucosinolates mix with enzymes in your saliva and are converted into chemicals called isothiocyanates and indole-3-carbinol. Now before you start wondering if you've enrolled in a biochemistry class, I promise we'll keep the science part of the explanation as basic as possible. The key point to remember is that it's the *breakdown products* of the vegetables that are important.

In addition to glucosinolates, cruciferous vegetables also contain folic acid, vitamin C, potassium, selenium along with other phytochemicals (plant chemicals) such as chlorophyll, carotenoids, lignans and phytosterols. Please look at a serving of Brussels sprouts with respect the next time it's served to you!

What does this mean to you and our former President? The studies are exciting. The high percentage of glucosinolates in broccoli and the other vegetables in this family appear to have three important functions: (1) they help your liver remove toxins and potential cancer-causing chemicals from your body; (2) they help prevent normal cells from being turned into cancer cells; and (3) they help to alter the way we break down and remove hormones from our bodies in ways that may decrease the development of hormone-sensitive cancers such as breast or prostate cancer.

As you can imagine, it's hard to do research on big populations of people and nutrition. Most of the studies are done retrospectively. In other words, these studies rely on the participants' ability to recall their diets over the last weeks, months and years. In addition, we are beginning to understand that our individual genetic make-up has a huge impact on our cancer risks. In other words, some of us will benefit from having cruciferous vegetables in our diet more than others will. So where are the data leading? It looks as if people who consume more cruciferous vegetables will have a lower risk of both lung cancer and colon cancer. (Although smoking cessation will do more for your lung cancer risk than eating a plate full of broccoli!)

Cruciferous vegetables may also affect breast cancer rates (Rogan, 2003). We'll review the details in a later chapter on menopause.

So how many cruciferous vegetables should we eat? Does it matter how we prepare it? Dr. Eleanor Rogan of the Eppley Cancer Institute associated with the University of Nebraska Medical Center showed that there were fewer nutrients in microwaved broccoli than when it was steamed or roasted in the oven. For this reason, my colleagues and I recommend either steaming the vegetables or roasting the vegetables in a 450 degree oven. Tossing them with a small amount of olive oil and a little salt and pepper is also good. (Try roasting Brussels sprouts. When the outer leaves get brown and crunchy while the inside is sweet and soft, you may change your mind about these little vegetables!)

The National Cancer Institute is recommending that we eat five to nine servings of fruits and vegetables a day; we suggest five servings of cruciferous vegetables a week. And, of course, the next time a President complains about a cruciferous vegetable, you'll know what to say!

Organic Thoughts

We're blessed in America to have a wide array of fruits and vegetables to choose from in the grocery store. Thanks to greenhouses, the trucking industry and huge agricultural businesses, we see produce year-round in our supermarkets. In addition to the wide selection, we are seeing the terms *organically grown* or *commercially grown*. Some stores are listing the country or state of origin so we can decide if we want cherries from Chile or peaches from Georgia in our shopping decisions. In 2002 the USDA issued a new series of labels to give the agricultural industry guidelines regarding the use of the term *organic*.

The Organic Foods Production Act (OFPA) and the National Organic Program (NOP) have developed labeling requirements that apply to raw, fresh products and processed products that contain organically grown ingredients. The federal standards are meant to apply to everyone except operations whose gross annual income from sales is $5,000 or less. There is a penalty of $11,000 levied if a manufacturer knowingly sells or labels a product that is not produced and handled in accordance with the NOP regulations.

Organic agricultural products are labeled either "100 percent organic," "organic" or "made with organic ingredients." A label that says "100 percent organic" means just what the name says. All of the ingredients must be organic. The FDA excludes water and salt in the processing, but every other processing aid and ingredient must be grown and processed organically. The items cannot be produced using sewage sludge or ionizing radiation.

The term *organic* implies the product consists of at least 95 percent organically produced ingredients, again excluding water and salt. Similar to the 100 percent organic product, the items cannot be produced using sewage sludge or ionizing radiation. The FDA has a National List that includes specific nonorganically produced agricultural products that are not currently commercially available in organic form. If an item is "organic," than the rest of the ingredients must come from the FDA's National List.

A product that is labeled "made with organic ingredients," on the other hand, is saying that at least 70 percent of the ingredients are organic. Processed foods can list up to three of the ingredients on the label. (For example a soup can be labeled either "made with organic peas, potatoes and carrots" or "made with organic vegetables.") Products with this labeling again cannot be produced using sewage sludge or ionizing radiation.

If a processed product has less than 70 percent organic ingredients, the manufacturer cannot use the term *organic* on the label. They can, however, itemize which ingredients are organically grown.

So why does this matter? More than one study has compared fruits and vegetables that were grown organically versus commercially. For example, a Rutgers study in the 1990s compared commercially grown produce to organic produce and noted a marked difference in nutritional value. The products themselves have been bred to look nice in the store and have a long shelf life; nutritional concerns are often secondary. Another study in Pennsylvania grew oats and wheat in the same field and used organic techniques on half of the plants and pesticides and other commercial cultivation procedures on the other half. The organically grown wheat had 16 percent higher protein than the commercially grown wheat, 108 percent higher vitamin B1, 131 percent higher vitamin B2 and 63 percent higher niacin. Calcium was 29 percent higher, and phosphorous was 1 percent higher in the organically grown wheat. There was a similar improvement in protein and nutrients in the organically grown oats.

When I encourage my patients to eat organic food, the frequent complaint is the higher cost to purchase organic food. Is the cost saving real for commercially grown food? Are we taking into account the contamination of ground water with pesticides? Agricultural pollutants have been found at both the north and south poles of the earth and can be detected in the deepest reaches of the oceans. There are studies that suggest pesticides may be causative culprits in Parkinson's disease in adults and autism in children.

Of course all fruits and vegetables should be washed before they are eaten. This is especially important for commercially grown produce. If there are "nooks and crannies" in fruits such as strawberries and raspberries, I strongly recommend organic produce only. Apples and cherries are best bought from organic growers only. If the skin is removed in order to eat the produce, such as a banana or an avocado, I still recommend washing the fruit thoroughly prior to eating them.

Most importantly, find the farms that use organic practices around you and support them! Community supported agricultural cooperatives are becoming more common. Your health and the health of your loved ones are worth it.

Sugar and Artificial Sweeteners: How Sweet It Is

Here's a not-so-nice statistic for you: the average American consumes 154 pounds of sugar per year. This amounts to more than 53 teaspoonfuls per person per day! Two researchers at the University of North Carolina at Chapel Hill reported that the percentage of total calories in our "average American diet" that comes from sugar, high-fructose corn syrup and other caloric sweeteners in the year 2000 was *32 percent higher* than it was in 1962. Their data suggest that the sugary calories are replacing calories from higher-fiber and more nutrient-dense foods.

It is clear that this high sugar load is the cause of the burgeoning problem of obesity, diabetes, high blood triglyceride levels, and low HDL (the good cholesterol) levels. Research also shows that excessive sugar causes an elevation in the stress hormone cortisol and other markers of inflammation such as C-reactive protein. What you may not know is that sugar in our bloodstream triggers the *same* "reward" response through the *same* neurochemical pathways that drug use does. So sugar is as addictive as heroin or crystal meth! Is there a 12-step program for sugar addiction? Well let's start with some education and empowerment.

A simple solution to limiting sugar in the diet is to avoid processed foods in the grocery store. As I said earlier, we like to encourage our clients to stay out of the middle of the grocery store.

If you find yourself in one of the middle aisles, however, read the label of the product you're considering and avoid buying foods that have sugar as one of the first three ingredients. Watch out also for other sugar "disguises" such as high-fructose corn syrup, sucrose, glucose, maltose, dextrose, lactose, fructose, corn syrup, or white grape juice concentrate. Also watch for honey, barley malt, maple sugar, sucanat, natural cane sugar, and dehydrated cane juice.

I'm frequently asked about artificial sweeteners. There's a huge assortment in the sugar bowl—do you get confused with the different colored packets? Let me see if I can clear up the confusion and make some rational suggestions.

Artificial sweeteners or sugar substitutes are compounds that offer the sweetness of sugar without the same number of calories. They are anywhere from 30 to 8,000 times sweeter than sugar. Ira Remsen developed the first artificial sweetener in 1879 at Johns Hopkins University. He accidentally spilled a chemical on his hand (and tasted it? This is usually not encouraged in chemistry labs!), and it was ultimately developed into saccharin (Sweet-n-Low, which is the pink packet on the table). The FDA tried to ban saccharine in 1977 because of animal studies that showed an increased risk of cancer with its use. The food industry intervened by lobbying Congress, and the sweetener was kept on the market with a warning label.

Another sweetener is aspartame (under the brand names of NutraSweet or Equal—the blue packets on the table), which is a combination of two amino acids (phenylalanine and aspartic acid). The safety of aspartame has been under debate. Of one hundred sixty-six studies on aspartame, seventy-four had at least partial food industry–related funding, and ninety-two were independently funded. While 100 percent of the industry-funded studies concluded aspartame is safe, 92 percent of the independently funded research identified potential problems such as a disruption in brain chemistry, depression and headaches. The only agreed-upon danger of aspartame is in people with phenylketonuria or PKU. People with PKU can't metabolize phenylalanine and should avoid aspartame completely.

The yellow packet on the table is sucralose or Splenda. This is the first artificial sweetener that is not affected by heat and can be used in baked goods and hot beverages. There are no long-term independent studies on the safety of sucralose to date.

Sugar alcohol sweeteners such as sorbitol, mannitol and xyolitol are frequently found in food. They are not absorbed but can cause abdominal gas, bloating and abdominal pain in large doses.

Already approved as a food additive and as a sweetener is glycyrrhizin, an extract of licorice root that is fifty to one hundred times sweeter than sucrose. Stevioside (under the brand name Stevia) comes from leaves of a South American plant and is three hundred times sweeter than sucrose. Dihydrochalcones (DHCs) are noncaloric sweeteners derived from bioflavonoids of citrus fruits that are approximately three hundred to two thousand times sweeter than sucrose.

I can absolutely guarantee that the food industry is going to continue to pursue the development and marketing of foods with artificial sweeteners. The financial payoff of a chemical that feeds our sugar addiction safely is their incentive.

The problem with this approach is that eating foods with artificial sweeteners does not cure sugar cravings. Some studies that looked at this found that subjects tended to eat *more* sugar-containing foods when they had high quantities of artificial sweeteners in their diets (Swithers, 2008).

All this leads me to suggest the following: Eat real food. Not cloned food. Not genetically modified food. Not processed food. Use artificial sweeteners very rarely or not at all. Recognize your sugar addiction. (It is worse for some of us than others!) Reach for a piece of fresh fruit or perhaps a cup of herbal tea when the craving hits. Remove high-sugar snacks from the house and learn what time of day is the hardest for you. (Right after work when I'm fixing dinner is mine!) Like all the 12-step programs say: get support with your addiction and take it one day at a time.

Good Fats: Something Fishy Is Going On

In the 1980s a National Institutes of Health conference announced that all Americans except children under two years of age should reduce their dietary fat from 40 percent to 30 percent of their daily diet to prevent heart disease. This started a "fat is bad" craze as the NIH suggested that we count fat grams and reduce fat in our diet. Walter Willett, the chairman of the Department of Nutrition at Harvard's School of Public Health, disparagingly called this "the SnackWell revolution" because the "low fat" cookies made by Nabisco exemplified this trend.

(As an aside, if you remember the previous section in this book on sugar, you'll know why I don't recommend eating SnackWell cookies. Here's the ingredient list from their Web site (the emphasis is mine): SnackWell, Ingredients: *sugar*, enriched flour, *high fructose corn syrup*, skim milk, cocoa, glycerin, emulsifiers, leavening, gelatin, cornstarch, modified corn starch, chocolate, salt, potassium sorbate added to preserve freshness, artificial flavor.)

Today, of course, we know that sugar and carbohydrate calories instead of fat calories are not better or healthier. Dr.

Willett notes that forty-four million people are now clinically obese compared with thirty million a decade ago. Heart disease is increasing in incidence, as is adult-onset diabetes and high blood pressure. Thanks to several large research studies we can now dispel the "fat is bad" message and change it to "there are good fats and bad fats." By the end of this section you will have some guidelines and recommendations on how to incorporate the good fats.

Two terms come up frequently when discussing good fats: *essential fatty acids* or EFAs and *polyunsaturated fatty acids* or PUFAs. PUFAs are the broad category of fatty acids that include the EFAs and their breakdown products. "Essential" means just what it says—these fats are essential for life. We can't manufacture them but must consume them as food or supplements. EFAs are the building blocks of our cell membranes—they allow nutrition into our cells and support receptors that allow each cell to communicate with other cells. The breakdown products of EFAs also modulate our response to inflammation. These fats could easily be the most important food or supplements in your diet.

EFAs are grouped into chemically similar subgroups based on where a carbon double bond appears in the long chain of carbons. Omega-3 fatty acids have the double bond at the third carbon in the chain, and omega-6 fatty acids have it at the sixth carbon in the chain. Most of us get plenty of the omega-6 EFAs from our diets. Vegetables, nuts and seeds all have omega-6 fats in them and so does chicken and beef. The average American diet has an average ratio of 20:1 of omega-6 to omega-3 fats. A more optimal ratio would be 3:1. Rather than cutting out the healthy omega-6 fats, we recommend supplementing omega-3 fats either nutritionally or with supplements.

Cold-water fatty fish have high levels of omega-3 fats. Examples include anchovies, bluefish, carp, catfish, halibut, herring, mackerel, pompano, salmon, tuna and whitefish. Plant-derived sources of omega-3 fats include walnuts, flaxseed oil (not capsules) and canola oil. Eating fish frequently is problematic for residents of the Midwest. Not only are we land-locked, but the potential for dioxins, polychlorinated biphenyls (PCBs) and methyl mercury contaminants in the coldwater fatty fish (especially the farm-raised fish) are worrisome. Because of this, the Food and Drug Administration has suggested that pregnant women limit their consumption of fish to twice a week and to limit themselves to "lower-risk" fish. An excellent Web site to review is www. environmentaldefense.org (search eco-friendly fish).

The American College of Obstetricians and Gynecologists recommends the following:

"Fish and shellfish are good sources of high-quality protein and other nutrients. However, pregnant women should not eat certain kinds of fish because they contain high levels of a form of mercury that can be harmful to the developing fetus. You should avoid eating shark, swordfish, king mackerel, or tilefish during pregnancy. These large fish contain high levels of mercury. Albacore tuna also is high in mercury so you may want to choose canned chunk light tuna instead. Other types of fish are fine in limited amounts. You can eat up to 12 ounces (two to three meals) of other varied fish and shellfish per week."

Dosing omega-3 fats should be based on the amount of two fats in particular: EPA (eicosapentaenoic acid) and DHA (docosahexaenoic acid). We recommend a minimum of 2 grams of EPA and DHA combined. Further, we prefer to work with companies that chelate out mercury and other toxins and also test each batch of fish oil capsules for strength and purity. We adjust the dose if our clients have arthritis or irritable bowel disease and if they're on blood thinners or anticoagulants. We suggest that our clients who are having surgery stop the supplemental fish oil two weeks before the surgery is scheduled. The FDA has stated that doses of fish oils up to 3 grams per day is generally regarded as safe. Higher doses may be associated with an increased risk of bleeding because fish oils appear to decrease platelet aggregation and prolong bleeding time, increase fibrinolysis (breaking down of blood clots), and may reduce von Willebrand factor.

The amounts of seafood necessary to provide one gram of the omega-3 two essential fats DHA and EPA (based on USDA Nutrient Data Laboratory information) is listed below:

- Pacific cod—23 ounces
- haddock—15 ounces
- catfish—15–20 ounces
- flounder/sole—7 ounces
- shrimp—11 ounces
- lobster—20 ounces
- sardines—3 ounces
- crab—8.5 ounces
- Atlantic cod—12.5 ounces
- clams—12.5 ounces
- scallops—17.5 ounces
- trout—3.5 ounces
- salmon—4.5 ounces
- herring—2 ounces
- oysters—4 ounces
- tuna (fresh)—6 ounces
- tuna (canned, light)—12 ounces

- tuna (canned, white)—4 ounces
- halibut—6 ounces
- mackerel—6 ounces
- cod liver oil—5 grams
- standard fish body oil—3 grams.

Omega-3 fats have been shown to reduce high triglyceride levels in the blood. The American Heart Association, in its 2003 recommendations, reports that supplementation with two ot four grams of omega-3 fats each day can lower triglycerides by 20 to 40 percent. These effects appear to be additive with "statin" drugs such as Lipitor. There are also studies that suggest omega-3 fats can decrease the incidence and severity of heart disease. There is a dose-related effect on high blood pressure with fish oil. Studies also show less inflammation in general and a decrease in the symptoms of rheumatoid arthritis, a decrease in the severity of irritable bowel disease, along with improved bronchial asthma and psoriasis. Omega-3 fats may also help decrease the risk of dialysis graft failure and assist with the recovery from organ transplants.

Exercising Options for Health

If we could give every individual the right amount of nourishment and exercise, not too little and not too much, we would have found the safest way to health.

Hippocrates

Those who think they have no time for bodily exercise will sooner or later have to find time for illness.

Edward Stanley

According to a review article by Canadian researcher Darren Warburton (2006), 51 percent of Canadians are physically inactive. (The American percentage is similar.) He reported that physical inactivity or lack of exercise is the biggest modifiable risk factor for heart disease, diabetes, cancer, high blood pressure, osteoporosis and arthritis. In other words, not exercising is riskier than smoking, riskier than alcohol or drug abuse, and riskier than anything else we choose to do (or not do) to optimize or challenge our health. Studies show that if we increase our physical activity even a little bit, then our risks of heart disease and diabetes are reduced.

Physically inactive middle-aged women who exercise less than one hour per week have a 52 percent increase in all-cause mortality, double their cardiovascular-related mortality, and have a 29 percent increase in cancer-related mortality compared with physically active women. The effect on health is graded—in other words, even slight increases in fitness or activity patterns show large improvements in our health and decrease the incidence of premature death.

The medical literature is full of articles on the benefits of exercise in reducing heart disease and blood vessel damage. There are articles on modifying blood sugar and blood lipid patterns with exercise. There are articles on reducing the incidence of breast and colon cancer with regular exercise. And the list goes on. The point is that the studies have been done on just about every health challenge you can think of, and the addition of moderate exercise improves the outcome each time. So why don't 51 percent of us exercise?

One factor that interferes with our exercise habits is television (Bennett, 2006). We know that we as Americans watch on average three to four hours of television daily. We also know that for every hour of television we watch, we walk one hundred forty-four fewer steps per day. (Do you have a pedometer? It's an excellent way to monitor activity level. The goal is ten thousand steps every day.) So one solution for increasing exercise is to turn off the television. Ditto the video games or the Internet. Trust me, there will be plenty of time for tweets and Facebook updates.

Another factor is our community. If there are no sidewalks to walk on or if safety is a concern in our neighborhood, then we won't choose to walk anywhere. Also, if our communities are developed and designed so that we need a car to get to the store or the bank, then we've lost some of our motivation to run our errands on bike or on foot.

The third reason we don't exercise is one of habit. If we don't exercise regularly and make it part of our daily/weekly life, it doesn't happen. Our schedules intervene. A meeting comes up; we stay late at work. Some people solve the scheduling issue by choosing to buy a gym membership or signing up with a personal trainer. This is a financial commitment to health and your monthly check nudges you to get your money's worth from the investment. I have friends who exercise at a "boot camp" at the crack of dawn every weekday before work. The schedule is grueling, but after committing to and completing one session of a few months, their stamina is improved, they've lost weight, and they feel sharper mentally. I should also mention that regular exercise is a great way to increase libido. In addition, a regular exercise program raises serotonin and is an excellent treatment for anxiety and depression.

If your budget doesn't allow a personal trainer or a gym membership, there are less expensive (and free) habits for exercise. You can use the stairs instead of the elevator whenever possible. You can park at the far end of the parking lot whenever you go out to eat or to the mall. You can stop at that park on the way home with the walking track and walk a few laps. You can pick up an exercise video and make a commitment to work out with it every day.

The ideal exercise program has a combination of exercise that increases your heart rate such as walking, cycling or swimming. In addition, it includes some type of muscle toning or strengthening such as yoga, Pilates, weight machines or exercise bands. And guess what? It should be enjoyable. Exercise shouldn't feel like a punishment or penance! Talk a friend into walking with you. Change the venue to a "mall walk" on stormy days. The key to exercise success is consistency. Commit to three twenty-minute walks a week; your health is worth the effort.

2

Stress Management

The Merriam-Webster dictionary defines stress as "a physical, chemical, or emotional factor that causes bodily or mental tension and may be a factor in disease causation." The work of the Austrian physician Hans Selye set the stage for our current exploration of the effect of stress on our health. As we unlock the human genome, more and more information is flooding in on the effect of stress on aging, weight gain, cancer growth, depression and more. Practically every type of therapy in integrative medicine is modifying the effect of stress on our physical, emotional, mental and spiritual health.

Fear, Stress and Anxiety, Oh My!

These are challenging times. I wrote this line as the November 2008 election was lurching to an end, the financial markets were restructuring before our eyes and our area here in the Midwest was reeling from a ferocious windstorm that left many of us without power for almost a week. Each of these in isolation would be unsettling or anxiety provoking—taken together they can unground and shift us way out of energetic and physical balance. So let's look at how this is engaging our energy and explore strategies for coming back into our optimal balance. We'll begin with awareness and assessment and then finish with energetic tools and strategies to remember and apply.

How do we know that we're stressed? It's important to remember that the ability to respond to stress is actually a good thing. We can all think of times when being focused, alert and responsive was crucial to survival. If we're driving on a highway in heavy traffic, for example, or operating a chain saw, or negotiating a business deal—these are all times where increased awareness and focus are absolutely essential. Our bodies are amazingly capable of sensing potential danger and responding immediately; our sympathetic nervous system kicks in and releases adrenaline, norepinephrine and cortisol. These neurotransmitters flood our body and cause our heart rate to increase so it can pump more oxygen to our brain and cause our blood sugar to go up and give us a short-term jolt of energy.

Ideally, we respond to stress and then relax back to a normal state. In reality, the stress hormones continue to flow in many people. This continuous release of stress hormones results in many symptoms. Warning signs of stress include such diverse signs and symptoms as memory problems, indecisiveness, increased anxiety or worry, agitation, irritability, sadness, muscle tension, headaches or backaches, frequent infections, drug and alcohol abuse, and changes in eating and sleeping habits. We all respond to stress slightly differently. Assessing our own individual warning signs are tremendously important. We need to be able to recognize how our life stressors play out in our body, mind and spirit. Research shows that most diseases are worsened by the presence of stress.

After awareness, the next step is to reach for tools that can "unwind" our stress pattern. One tool is to reframe our awareness of the problem. My friend Mackey McNeill is a CPA whose newsletter recently gave a great summary of the financial crisis (www.cultivatingprosperity.com). She notes that bear markets last an average of 14.7 months and this is the eleventh bear market since World War II. I learned that we are twelve months into this bear market and markets move upward at the height of pessimism. She also noted that our current economic challenge is primarily one of confidence.

Reading her words helped me see my own financial worries and anxiety in perspective. She added a depth to my understanding and helped me see the patterns of response that the financial markets can show. Think of people in your life who add balance to your perspective. Listen to their information and opinions and see if it adds dimension or a new way of looking at your concerns.

Another tool to use is bodywork such as massage or craniosacral therapy. Both techniques help unwind muscle tension. Combine them with a daily relaxation guided imagery CD or meditation or quiet prayer and see if your pattern of response shifts to one with less pain or anxiety.

My favorite tool in the toolbox is a combination of chiropractic adjustment, acupuncture and energy work. We term this an "ACE" where I work—and it is an efficient and enjoyable way to return to emotional, physical and spiritual balance.

A walk outside can make a difference. Walk quietly with the conscious connection and awareness of your feet in your shoes on the earth. Tune in to the colors and textures and smells around you. Practice a "spirit walk"—walk slow enough that you breathe in when you step on your right foot and breathe out when you step on your left foot. Repeat this for a few minutes and notice how your tension eases as your breathing literally slows you down.

Focus on gratitude as a conscious choice every day. Think of perhaps three things every day (or every hour) for which you're grateful. At the moment, looking out my window, I'm grateful for the bright red male cardinal on the bush outside. I'm grateful for a warm, dry place to write. Looking at the picture of my loved ones on my desk, I'm grateful I was born into a loving and supportive family. Try it! A practice of gratitude is easy to do—maybe write it down for the first month—then watch your life transform.

Finding Light in the Darkness—Seasonal Affective Disorder

We all know that time of year when we sense the onset of winter. The blanket of leaves in the yard appears almost overnight, and the crisp morning air reminds me of the next season waiting in the wings. The birds outside my window have fluffed up their down jackets against the cold. And there's more darkness. As our days shorten, we're more likely to leave for work in the dark and drive home after work in the dark. We know intuitively that this cycle of light and dark happens every year—why does it catch us off guard? What's triggering the regret and sadness as winter comes?

Seasonal affective disorder (SAD) is a type of depression that affects half a million people in the U.S. every winter, with a peak incidence in December, January and February. Three out of four SAD people are women with the main age of onset between eighteen and thirty. It is rare to develop SAD within 30 degrees of the equator, and it can occur in either the northern or southern hemisphere. Now we're starting to understand more about the reason for these "winter blues."

Buried in the base of the brain is the pineal gland, which produces a hormone or chemical messenger called melatonin. In the animal kingdom, the pineal gland controls circadian rhythms such as when to sleep, when to wake, when to migrate, when to hibernate, when to build a nest and become pregnant or lay eggs. Now there are data to show that melatonin plays a role in temperature regulation, the function of the immune system and even the onset of sexual maturity in the animal kingdom.

But what of humans? Prior to fifty years ago, the pineal gland was thought to be a vestigial or remnant organ without significant function. (Similar to the appendix attached to the large intestine—although we're starting to appreciate the role of the appendix in "re-seeding" the GI tract with beneficial bacteria after antibiotics are used.) Research has shown that melatonin is synthesized in our bodies from the neurotransmitter serotonin and that the levels of melatonin rise with the onset of darkness while the serotonin levels drop at night as it is turned into melatonin. Daylight is perceived by the retina in the back of our eyes, which sends a message to the pineal gland and "shuts down" melatonin production until the darkness returns.

Because of this research, many people have used melatonin supplements to help with sleep patterns; the problem with this approach is that melatonin probably doesn't cause the sleep cycle to "turn on" as much as it plays a part in inhibiting the brain's urge to be awake. In other words, perhaps the reason why not everyone benefits from using the supplement for improving sleep is that some other hormonal imbalance is causing the wakefulness.

As you can imagine, there is a lot of interest in understanding the human side of the pineal gland and melatonin story. For instance, we know that melatonin levels are high in children from ages four to seven and then levels decline overall—presumably to allow puberty to begin to develop. In addition, studies in mice show that the immune system is up-regulated in the presence of melatonin while antibody production is reduced if the pineal gland is removed. We don't know how this plays out in our own immune function.

So what does this mean for people with SAD? The solutions will be different for everyone. One option is to increase the amount of daylight or full-spectrum light you're exposed to in a day. Open the blinds and curtains, install skylights, and arrange your schedule to be outside in midday. Some companies sell full-spectrum lights to turn on for a period of time before or after daylight ends. Another option is to "migrate" south with the birds and spend the winter in sunnier climates. (Ohio in February can be twenty-eight days of gray—I recommend a break!)

Pay attention to the quality and quantity of food in your diet. Although it is harder to find fresh, locally grown organic produce in the Midwestern winter, perhaps you have frozen or canned some of your bountiful harvest and can turn to nourishing whole grains and soups and stews. Experiment with root vegetables and cold weather crops. Exercise daily. Bundle up and enjoy the lacy ice branches and the quiet snowscapes. Or commit to the gym and listen to a book on tape or that jazz CD you just bought as you work out.

Most of all, appreciate the changes in the light/dark cycle. Pay attention to the increase in the darkness as the days shorten until the winter solstice on or around December 21, and then celebrate the return of the light as then the days begin to lengthen again. It happens every year, yet we're caught up in the holiday "busy-ness" and often miss it.

3

The Integrative Medicine Toolbox

There are many tools in the integrative medicine toolbox. I've summarized some of the tools here that I've either used personally or witnessed their effectiveness. This chapter is by no means exhaustive; rather I've chosen examples that are widely available and reproducibly effective by most practitioners.

Acupuncture

President Richard Nixon's willingness to open diplomatic relations with China allowed the American ping-pong team to play in a tournament with the Chinese team in Beijing in 1971. This groundbreaking event was widely reported by the world press. Along with the sports and political reporting, a front-page article in the *New York Times* by staff writer James Reston described how he developed acute appendicitis during the tournament, how he was treated surgically by the local Chinese hospital staff and how his post-operative pain was managed by three strategically placed acupuncture needles. His article brought widespread public and professional awareness to acupuncture and traditional Chinese medicine. Training programs were set up as the Western medical community explored and experimented with Eastern medicine treatments. There was a search to understand why acupuncture worked, and in the 1970s there was no shortage of technology to apply to the question.

Unlike in the United States, in Europe there had been a quiet but steady exploration of Eastern medicine. Jesuit missionaries in the sixteenth and seventeenth centuries brought back stories from China and coined the term *acupuncture* from the Latin *acus* (needle) and *punctura* (puncture). They described pulse diagnosis, medicinal herbs and teas and the acupuncture treatments. French physicians in Indochina brought back information in the mid-nineteenth century, as did the French diplomat George Soulie de Morant. He published the first European text on acupuncture in the mid-twentieth century based on Chinese and Japanese articles and texts.

The oldest Chinese text is the *Huang Di Nei Jing (Yellow Emperor's Inner Classic)*, which was compiled in the era of the Han dynasty (206 BC to 220 AD) The *Nei Jing* describes the human body in the context of the universe; both Confucianism (the correct manner of human co-existence in society) and Daoism (the balance of nature in a medical context) are included in its writings.

The Chinese believe we are balanced energetically between heaven and earth. Using energy super-highways, or meridians, their writings say our energy or "chi" (also spelled "qi") travels up through our bodies from earth to heaven and back down from heaven to earth. All of our bodily functions such as breathing, digestion, circulation, reproduction and menstruation are balanced by this flow of energy throughout the organs and the body.

In this framework, think of disease as an imbalance or a blockage of the energy flow. An example is a stream that gets blocked by a rock or fallen tree as debris and clutter build up on the stream bed, forcing the water to flow in a different pattern or more slowly through the blockage. A Traditional Chinese Medicine practitioner prescribes acupuncture, nutritional therapies and exercises to increase energy flow to the area of blockage. Acupuncture needles are placed in strategic points to open up the blockages in energy. A typical session lasts about thirty to sixty minutes.

There is now a large body of research on acupuncture. There are brain imaging studies. Tissue culture studies explore local response to acupuncture, and double-blind studies use placebo needles that prove effectiveness in areas such as pain management, fertility and menopausal symptoms.

I am a student of acupuncture through Joseph Helms, MD, an iconic character in the training of physicians through the Helms Medical Institute, affiliated with UCLA. Dr. Helms has written a textbook *Acupuncture Energetics* and a book for the lay audience called *Getting to Know You* (Helms, 2007) and has trained thousands of physicians. He practices acupuncture and internal medicine in southern California and brings a dynamic and intelligent organization to the study of acupuncture. I am indebted to him and the preceptors in his training course who shared their knowledge and skills.

Acupuncture remains one of the treatments that I do every day I practice medicine. I am blessed because I am encouraged and allowed to use acupuncture in a balanced and energetic context. There is no doubt in my mind that acupuncture can significantly help most medical conditions. The World Health Organization recommends acupuncture for the following conditions:

Respiratory Diseases
- Acute sinusitis
- Acute rhinitis
- Common cold
- Acute tonsillitis

Bronchopulmonary Diseases
- Acute bronchitis
- Bronchial asthma

Eye Disorders
- Acute conjuctivitis
- Cataract (without complications)
- Myopia
- Central retinitis

Disorders of the Mouth Cavity
- Toothache
- Pain after tooth extraction
- Gingivitis
- Pharyngitis

Orthopedic Disorders
- Tennis elbow
- Sciatica
- Low back pain
- Rheumatoid arthritis

Gastrointestinal Disorders
- Spasm of the esophagus and cardia
- Hiccups
- Gastroptosis
- Acute and chronic gastritis
- Gastric hyperacidity
- Chronic duodenal ulcer
- Acute and chronic colitis

- Acute bacterial dysentery
- Constipation
- Diarrhea
- Paralytic ileus
  Neurologic Disorders
- Headache
- Migraine
- Trigeminal neuralgia
- Facial paralysis
- Paralysis after apoplectic fit
- Peripheral neuropathy
- Paralysis caused by polio
- Meniere's syndrome
- Neurogenic bladder dysfunction
- Nocturnal enuresis
- Intercostal neuralgia

Energy Medicine—Healing Touch, Reiki

Many of my patients talk about their energy levels. They're not talking about levels of fossil fuels or exploring sustainable carbon neutral technologies. They're talking about fatigue or energy depletion. Western medicine evaluates fatigue and low energy by ruling out conditions such as anemia, underactive thyroid and infections such as mononucleosis, among others. Functional medicine testing can add a layer of nuance to the assessment by actually measuring the efficiency of cellular energy and explore nutritional deficiencies or toxic exposures.

On the other hand, my Eastern medical training explores a broader focus—what's going on emotionally, mentally, spiritually as well as physically. Integrative medicine includes less traditional therapies that we group in the category of energy medicine. We use this term for any healing modality that works by contacting and moving energy within the body. Types of energy medicine include healing touch, Reiki, craniosacral therapy and energy movement exercises such as Tai Chi and Qi Gong.

Janet Mentgen, RN, BSN, developed healing touch as a continuing education program for nurses in 1989. The program is taught in several levels and draws on teachings and writings of energy healers that include Barbara Brennan, Alice Bailey and Rosalyn Bruyere. Hands are placed on or near the body allowing the flow of energy to be redirected and promoting a feeling of deep relaxation. Its goal is to restore the body's natural flow of energy, thus facilitating self-healing. Healing touch is complementary to other health care modalities.

Reiki is a Japanese word meaning "universal life-force energy." The "ki" part of the word is the same word as Chi or Qi, the Chinese word for the energy that underlies every living thing. Reiki is a system for channeling life force energy to and through the practitioner's hands for the purpose of healing. Dr. Mikao Usui described Reiki healing in the early 1900s. He taught and traveled throughout Japan at the time, and during his travels he met Dr. Chujiro Hayashi, a Commander in the Naval Reserve. They traveled around Japan together teaching and healing and established a training program in Tokyo.

Mrs. Hawayo Takata was born in Hawaii, on Kauai, on Christmas Eve 1900 of Japanese descent. She was introduced to the healing power of Reiki in the 1930s when visiting her sister in Japan and popularized the technique in the United States after the Second World War. Reiki practitioners here in America learn the technique from other Reiki practitioners known as Reiki Masters.

Claudia E. Harsh, MD

Craniosacral Therapy

Dr. William Sutherland was in his senior year of osteopathic school in the early 1900s when he realized that the bones of the human skull were not fixed but capable of subtle movement. Although most Western countries did not recognize cranial motion, this possibility was not new to other cultures. Cranial manipulation has been practiced in India for centuries and was also developed by the ancient Egyptians and members of the Paracus culture in Peru (2000 BC to 200 AD). Furthermore, in the eighteenth century, the philosopher and scientist Emmanuel Swedenborg described a rhythmic motion of the brain, stating that it moves with regular cycles of expansion and contraction. Dr. Sutherland continued to study cranial manipulation and developed a training program for osteopaths in the 1930s that is still taught today.

Dr. John Upledger continued the research on cranial manipulation after observing the pulsation of the covering of the brain during a brain surgery in the mid-1970s. He studied the phenomenon and developed a teaching program for practitioners. Since he included nonosteopaths in the training, he coined the term *craniosacral therapy* to differentiate it from the cranial osteopathy taught by Dr. Sutherland.

Craniosacral therapy can be used for general wellness and relaxation as a preventive tool. My clients with migraine headaches, stress, anxiety, depression, pelvic pain, back pain and hypertension have had excellent results with regular craniosacral therapy treatments.

Guided Imagery and Health

True confessions: I don't like winter much. It's right about the middle of January after the holidays have ended that the stretch of gray winter days and frigid temperatures combine to turn my mind and heart toward spring. As I write this, I'm imagining the azalea bush outside my window teeming with pink blossoms, the woods filling with bright green new leaves and the return of the robins and the swarms of brown finches. If I focus long enough, I can remember the feeling of sunlight on my skin, the smell of hyacinths, the growling sputter of the lawnmower next door or any of a number of spring sensory memories.

These images are an important winter coping strategy for me (and, hey, if you need it, feel free to borrow it!). I can put on a piece of music that reminds me of spring (at the moment it's a Bach Brandenburg concerto) and take a mental break from my normal thoughts. This type of imagery is used extensively in integrative medicine, and there are more and more scientific studies to support its use.

Guided imagery is a technique that uses music and a series of verbal suggestions and affirmations to achieve a progressive relaxation of the body and mind. There are excellent CDs available on a large number of topics including both acute and chronic pain, cancer treatment side effects, smoking cessation, menopausal hot flashes and fertility, just to name a few. I recommend its use to nearly every new patient I see; I believe this technique is easy to practice, relatively inexpensive and remarkably free of untoward side effects. Having said that, however, I hasten to add that imagery is only a tool, and even though it is widely applicable, it is not always a substitution for pharmaceutical drugs or surgery if indicated. I've listed here a few studies just to give you a snapshot of current research efforts.

Researchers in Brazil used relaxation and guided imagery in patients with breast cancer who were getting radiation therapy (Nunes, 2007). Half of the patients had routine care, while the other half had a group relaxation session for twenty-four consecutive days while they were in for their radiation therapy. Clinical interviews showed lower amounts of stress, anxiety and depression in the group that had the imagery and relaxation sessions. Cortisol levels were lower in the clients with less stress although the researchers added that there was no measured effect on the immune system.

Migraine headaches were studied in India; a randomized controlled trial where half of the enrolled patients used systematic relaxation with abdominal breathing and a beta blocker (propranolol) in the other half (Kaushik, 2005). The two groups were followed for six months. The two groups had similar responses including a decrease in frequency, severity and the duration of migraine attacks. However, a year after the study was concluded, there was a significantly lower number of recurrent headaches in the group that had been exposed to the relaxation training.

At Cedars-Sinai in Los Angeles a group of patients with stable coronary heart disease were split into two groups—one group had their routine sixteen-week health education program, and the other group was taught a relaxation tool called Transcendental Meditation (TM) (Paul-Labrador, 2006). Interestingly enough, the TM group had lower systolic blood pressure and less insulin resistance. The next step of research is to look at long-term health outcomes for differences.

There have been eighteen studies of surgery patients, according to one review article. Compared to patients who did not practice the guided imagery before and during surgery, the imagery patients had lower amounts of blood loss, less anxiety, a shorter hospital stay and used a lower amount of pain medication after surgery (Blankfield, 1991).

Duke University is currently working with the Department of Veterans Affairs to research the effect of guided imagery on post-traumatic stress disorder (PTSD). Several pilot studies have suggested that this is going to be an extremely effective tool for people suffering from this problem.

I hope these examples intrigue you. What could you accomplish in your life if you turned the goal into an affirmation and used it in a regular guided imagery? You could survive the cold winter with thoughts of spring, as I do. You could stop smoking. You could release tension in your neck and shoulders and reduce headaches. You could reduce the frequency and intensity of hot flashes. Perhaps we could widen our imagery efforts to a countrywide or even a global effort? I'm ready; will you join me?

4

Understanding the Cycle of Life

The Conversation of Menarche

I was in sixth grade. All the sixth-grade girls in our public elementary school in South Carolina were taken to the auditorium for a "special conversation" while the boys were taken to a "special conversation" of their own in the gymnasium. I already knew about menstruation thanks to my mother and one of my older sisters. The atmosphere at school that day was tense. Girls were giggling and had facial expressions of amused disgust. Where an open and accepting attitude toward menstrual cycles could have been expressed, we had instead embraced the cultural norm. We were already aware of the cultural message that menstruation was dirty, painful and a hassle. The euphemisms for our cycles were telling: "the curse," "on the rag" or "the red plague."

Although my introduction from my mother was nonjudgmental and educational and the presentation at school was fact based, what I remember about that time was the extreme discomfort we felt as a group. And what about the boys in my sixth-grade class?

The very fact that they weren't included in our discussion made it clear this wasn't a topic for mixed company.

The normal age for menstruation to begin is between the ages of nine and sixteen with an average of 12.8 years. Most young women have the beginnings of breast development, pubic hair growth and a growth spurt before their cycles start, although *wide variations* exist. Gynecologists and pediatricians can answer questions about this if you're wondering about yourself or your loved ones.

But what causes our menstrual cycles to start? My sixth-grade brain asked that question and was given a one-word answer: *hormones.* Those amazingly powerful and mysterious hormones. We could be the victims of a surprise attack of these hormones at any time. (I didn't appreciate this lack of control over my own body!) I have heard many disparaging comments about hormones through my years as a gynecologist. A common question my patients asked was, "Is it me or is it my hormones?" with the implication that all would be right with their world if they could only get their hormones to toe the line and behave. In truth, we could no more live without our hormones than we could live without air! Moreover, our hormones are intimately involved in all aspects of cellular communication and growth.

I've come to reframe the conversation that my sixth-grade brain heard. Hormones are simply messages that are sent among organs in our body. Menstrual cycles start because of an intricate balance of hormonal cues or messages—and it all comes down to communication. Think of an e-mail between two people. The sender writes a message to the receiver. The receiver picks up the message and translates it and responds. This communication needs good clear *messages* and good clear lines of communication.

A *conversation* occurs when there are messages back and forth between the people.

Now translate this to a menstrual cycle. In this case, the part of the brain called the hypothalamus sends an e-mail to the pituitary, a small stalklike projection at the base of the brain. The pituitary responds with another e-mail message or hormone to the ovaries. When the ovaries receive the message, they turn back around and send another message—this time in the form of the hormones estrogen and progesterone in a cyclic wave. These messages signal the lining of the uterus to build up or break down over and over. When the lining of the uterus breaks down or sloughs, this results in a menstrual cycle. The length and amount of flow depends on how much of the lining was "built up" in the previous cyclic wave of hormone messages.

As in any conversation, there is room for a response to the message at every stage of the conversation—in medicine we call this feedback. So this means that the ovaries can "talk back" to the hypothalamus or the pituitary. Similarly, if there are other "conversations" going on in the body, they can change the way the lining of the uterus builds up and breaks down.

Let's think of some examples together.

Many people are aware that dancers or athletes who train hours on end and restrict their intake of calories can stop having menstrual cycles completely. Their body's e-mail messages are interrupting their normal hormonal conversation. The lining of the uterus gets different messages and stops its cyclic growth and release.

Another "interrupted conversation" example would be in times of stress and anxiety. During stressful times, the brain's conversation shifts from the ovary to the adrenal gland. Nobody can carry on conversations effectively with more than one person at a time. If your body is "paying more attention" to the stress hormone cortisol from the adrenal gland, then you can expect your ovaries are not making as much of their hormones estrogen and progesterone. The result here is an interruption of the cyclic hormonal messages to the uterine lining and a disruption of the menstrual cycle. This means the cycle could be shorter than normal, longer than normal, heavier than normal, lighter than normal … you get the idea.

If I understand that my menstrual cycle is a continuous conversation in my body among parts of my brain, my ovaries and my uterus, then it makes sense that variations in cycle length or cramps or other symptoms with the cycle arise from subtle changes in these conversations. If I appreciate that this hormonal conversation is an expression of the connection of my body to the world, then menstruation is not a curse or a plague; it's an indicator of balance. And this intricate balance of hormones can be interrupted by a change in nutrition, exercise level or stress. Where was that message in sixth grade? What can we do to change the cultural beliefs about menstruation?

Premenstrual Syndrome or PMS

Katharina Dalton in England coined the term *premenstrual syndrome* or PMS in the 1950s. She described the syndrome as a spectrum of symptoms that occur just before the menstrual cycle but then decrease in severity with the onset of menstrual bleeding. The symptoms can be emotional symptoms of irritability, fatigue and depression or physical symptoms of bloating, cramping or sugar cravings. My clinical experience is that PMS is very common, most women are affected to some degree. Researchers agree that symptoms are rare before the age of fourteen and usually disappear during pregnancy and menopause.

The psychiatric guide known as the DSM-IV (*Diagnostic and Statistical Manual of Mental Disorders, Fourth Edition*) published in the mid 1990s included a listing for a severe form of PMS called PMDD or premenstrual dysphoric disorder. In PMDD, the symptoms are still cyclic—occurring just before the menstrual cycle—and are marked by severe depression, a decreased interest in usual activities, lethargy or lack of energy, and either sleeping too much or too little.

Studies have shown a 60 percent improvement in severe PMS symptoms with the use of drugs such as sertraline (Zoloft), fluoxetine (Prozac, Sarafem) or other antidepressants. I don't argue that prescription options are occasionally necessary, but if PMS and PMDD are classified as mental illnesses, then we as women look for the solution *in a pill* rather than looking at the issue more holistically or culturally or globally.

Christiane Northrup, MD, is an ob-gyn from Yarmouth, Maine, who has a gift for educating and communicating with women about their bodies. She reframed the discussion of PMS and the menstrual cycles in terms of the moon and its phases (Northrup, 2006). The full moon is bright and shining with power and light. The new moon, on the other hand, is shrouded in darkness and mystery. Imagine, then, a typical woman with her responsibilities at home, at work and in her spiritual community. During mid-cycle she is outgoing, shining and giving freely of her time and energy. She is shining like the full moon with light and grace. Prior to her menstrual cycle she becomes more introspective and finds herself needing more "down time." If she honors that internal need, she'll spend more time resting or reading. If she "pushes through" the need and continues her usual schedule, she's likely to be more irritable or grouchy.

This is the most common scenario for a patient who asks me for a solution for PMS. Although she may complain of physical discomforts such as cramping, bloating or headaches, her main concern is her emotional lability, irritability and depression. Her family notices, of course, and she comes in asking for a fix. She doesn't necessarily want to hear my theories on hormonal communication and honoring the cycles of our bodies. She's accepted a cultural perspective on her menstrual cycle and feels her hormones are conspiring to ruin her life!

So how can we treat PMS? The first thing to do is to make sure of the diagnosis. This is best done with a diary; you chart your menstrual cycles and any symptoms throughout the month. Use a chart like the one here to note symptoms. Use the first row to write the dates using day number 1 as the first day of menstrual flow. Obviously the columns could be added to reflect your individual cycle length. Then use the chart to mark symptoms such as depression (place a D in the space under the date), irritability (place an I in the space under the date), breast discomfort (B), headache (H), a change in energy level (E), nausea (N) and so on. Place an X under each date when bleeding occurs and keep the diary for a few months. Watch the symptoms over a period of time—at least two or three months.

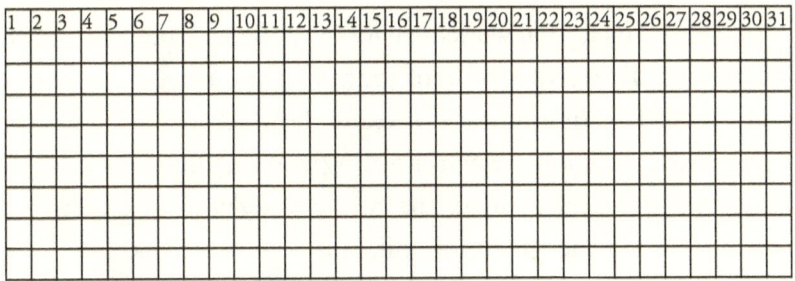

If the symptoms are cyclic and end with the menstrual cycle, it is probably PMS. Your clinician should rule out other potential causes of the symptoms such as a low blood count (anemia), depression, an underactive thyroid or hypoglycemia (abnormal sugar metabolism).

The two most important treatments for PMS are diet and exercise. In general it's best to avoid sugary foods and caffeine. A modified Mediterranean diet with lots of colorful organic vegetables, fruits, whole grains and chicken or fish is absolutely essential. Regular cardiovascular exercise can also reduce PMS symptoms dramatically. Just committing to a fifteen-minute walk three times a week will decrease many symptoms.

Some nutritional supplements can help PMS symptoms, including vitamin B6 or pyridoxine and vitamin E (with mixed tocopherols). Calcium and magnesium have been shown to help with PMS symptoms. Chaste tree (*Vitex agnus castus*) and cyclic progesterone cream can also be used, although controlled studies show mixed benefits overall. Your practitioner can evaluate your entire health history and your other medications for potential side effects that may be worsening your PMS symptoms.

Treatments that provide relaxation and raise your brain's serotonin levels such as massage therapy and acupuncture can also help PMS symptoms. Relaxation tapes, biofeedback treatments, meditation, yoga and Tai Chi will also make a difference.

One treatment that works well for my patients is proprioceptive journaling. To do this type of journaling you need a timer, a stereo with baroque music (for example, Bach or Vivaldi) and a pen and a notebook. Each morning you set the timer for ten to fifteen minutes, turn on the music and write as quickly as possible. When the timer goes off, close the notebook and don't read what you've written. You can also do this at a computer keyboard and then just delete the writing when the timer goes off. The idea of the journaling is to provide an emotional outlet; don't worry about spelling or syntax or grammar. This is meant to be a release valve for feelings like anger, frustration or sadness that are being stuffed down inside.

I encourage all women to look at the cultural "baggage" that we carry surrounding the menstrual cycle and reframe it into the cyclic wonder that it is. This cycle of life is a unique opportunity to stay awake and aware of our physical, emotional, mental and spiritual health. We're given a monthly fluctuation of hormones to practice awareness and balance. Honoring the cycle by caring for ourselves during the premenstrual portion of the cycle is the key.

Personal Growths: An Integrative Approach to Uterine Fibroids

By the time we're menopausal, as many as 75 to 80 percent of us will have at least one fibroid growth on our uterus. Fibroids are benign lumps of muscle and connective tissue in the uterus. They are very rarely found in girls before puberty and become more common as we age. African-American women are more likely to have fibroids than Caucasian women. Hormone therapy can cause existing fibroids to grow more rapidly. Depending on where the growths are located and how fast they're growing (if at all) will determine how symptomatic they are and whether or not they need to be removed. In general, fibroids will shrink in size with menopause.

Fibroids inside the uterine cavity or imbedded in the lining of the uterus can cause heavy menstrual bleeding—sometimes to the point of needing hospitalization and blood transfusion. On the other hand, if the fibroid is on the surface of the uterus, it may not even be noticeable except during a pelvic examination. Fibroids can grow quite large and can definitely cause pressure and pain in the abdomen. If the uterus feels larger than normal on examination, often doctors will start with an ultrasound or sonogram to measure the size and location of the fibroids. Fibroids are almost always benign (harmless). Because we can't tell if a tissue is benign without taking it out and looking at it under a microscope, close followup with exams and sonograms are important. The mere presence of fibroids doesn't mean that a hysterectomy is necessary. It does mean, however, that the fibroids should be followed closely.

If your fibroids are causing pain or excessive blood loss, then surgical treatment or hormonal treatments need to be done through your gynecologist. This section will talk about fibroids that are not necessarily causing severe problems but have been discovered on examination. We'll bring in a short discussion of acupuncture and Traditional Chinese Medicine and look at some interesting research on nutrition and mind-body medicine.

Traditional Chinese Medicine has evolved from techniques and theories that are thousands of years old. The Chinese believed that we are balanced energetically between heaven and earth. Using energy super-highways, or meridians, their writings say our energy or "chi" (also spelled "qi") travels up through our bodies from earth to heaven and back down from heaven to earth. All of our bodily functions—breathing, digestion, circulation and even menstruation are balanced by this flow of energy throughout the organs and the body. Think of fibroid tumors, then, as a disruption of energy flow—or a "stasis." A Traditional Chinese Medicine practitioner prescribes acupuncture, nutritional therapies and exercises to increase energy flow to the area.

Interestingly enough, a pilot study at the University of Arizona treated women with fibroids with weekly acupuncture, energy therapy, massage and guided imagery for six months. They compared these women with "controls"—women who were approximately the same age and with the same number of children and with the same size fibroids (Mehl-Madrona, 2002). Of the thirty-seven women in the treatment group, for twenty-two of them, their fibroids stopped growing or shrank and their bleeding decreased 72 percent. Only two of the women in the control group had this result. The authors comment that weekly treatments were more expensive than conventional medical therapies of surgery or pharmaceutical drugs and hormones. They note, however, that patient satisfaction was higher long term in the group treated with alternative therapies.

Another interesting study looked at nutrition in women with fibroids (Chiaffarino, 1999). A researcher in Italy interviewed women who had hysterectomies. Since he had the pathology reports, he could group the women into two groups: with and without fibroids. After interviewing the women, he reported that women with fibroids ate more beef and red meat and less fruits, vegetables and fish than women without fibroids.

Anecdotally, I know I saw more rapid fibroid growth in my patients who were in the midst of relationship difficulties. Whether it was marital problems, problems with their children or aging parents, I noted an increase in menstrual changes and fibroid growth. The energetic balance point or "chakra" over the uterine area is often called the relationship or second chakra. First described by yogis in the Hindu tradition, chakras are the meeting place of mind, body, emotions and soul. The second chakra is associated with desire, sensuality, procreation, pleasure, relationships, openness to others, creativity and empathy.

Questions to consider while journaling if you have fibroids would be these: Where do I feel stuck in my life? What is the fibroid telling me about how I might have blocked my energy or creativity? How can I free up my energy and live life more fully?

Integrating exercise, good nutrition and life balance with daily prayer, meditation or journaling is the key to keeping our energy flowing through our pelvis and uterus.

Ovarian Cysts and the CA-125 test

Because pelvic female anatomy is mostly hidden from view, pain can be difficult to diagnose correctly. Physicians rely on symptoms such as when the pain started, where it is located and what it feels like, along with what makes the pain better or worse. A pelvic exam can sometimes show if an infection is the cause of the pain or the suggestion of a mass or growth in the pelvis. Ultrasounds or sonograms can then confirm where the mass is located and if it is solid or cystic (fluid-filled) or a combination of both. In addition, the ultrasound can evaluate the rest of the pelvis.

Ovarian cysts are fluid-filled sacs within the ovary. Almost all ovarian cysts are benign (harmless). If an ultrasound has shown that you have an ovarian cyst (or cysts), more often than not your doctor will advise you to recheck the ultrasound after a menstrual cycle has passed. In addition, she may suggest that you have the recheck done while you're on your cycle before the next follicle starts to develop. As part of the normal "cycle of life" an egg grows within a cyst (called a follicle) until ovulation or egg release occurs. Because almost all women will have an ovarian cyst at some point in their cycle, let's focus our discussion on when the diagnosis is a potential concern.

If pelvic pain is present and an ovarian cyst is diagnosed, your first questions should be these: How big is the cyst? Where is it? Is it just one cyst (simple) or is the cyst complex (multiple cysts and solid areas)? Remember again that almost all ovarian cysts are benign. If the cyst persists and the pain persists, occasionally medicines or surgery are necessary. Most of the time the pain and the cyst resolve without intervention.

Even though I've said twice in the last three paragraphs that most ovarian cysts are benign, every time I see a patient with the diagnosis of an ovarian cyst, her biggest concern is ovarian cancer. Why is this? Because high-profile actresses like Gilda Radner died at a young age of ovarian cancer? Or perhaps because the symptoms of ovarian cancer are nonspecific and vague?

I believe that even though the disease is rare (1.4 to 2.5 percent of women will get ovarian cancer), there is a mindset of fear in our culture. There is fear of death, fear of pain, fear of medical expenses, fear of terrorist attack, fear of ... well you get the idea! For this reason, I am frequently asked about using the CA-125 blood test as a screening for ovarian cancer. This is almost always *not* a good idea.

In order to be a good screening test, the results of the test should be positive when cancer is present and negative when it isn't. Although the CA-125 test can be used to follow the *treatment* of ovarian cancer, elevated levels are not always found when cancer is present. Perhaps more worrisome, an elevated level in a woman without a cancer diagnosis is almost always not cancer. (Estimates are that when used as a screening tool, as many as 96 percent of abnormally high CA-125 tests are not because of cancer. Any abdominal irritation including endometriosis or irritable bowel syndrome can cause an elevation in the CA-125 test.)

Acupuncture, gentle pelvic massage, castor oil packs and pelvic physical therapy can all be used to help resolve ovarian cysts. Close communication and follow-up with your gynecologist are important. If the pain worsens or the cyst persists or increases in size, it's appropriate to intervene with medicines or surgery or both.

While waiting and watching, the integrative therapies can be used. In this situation, I find that acupuncture can serve several purposes: it can help move stuck energy or qi through the pelvis. Similar to the treatment of fibroids or endometriosis, the acupuncture needles are placed in the arms, legs, abdomen and head to move and balance energy. It can also help with relaxation and anxiety. When used in conjunction with a regular journaling practice, acupuncture can help reveal the reasons for fear, and we can explore strategies for coping with or understanding the fear. If fear is acknowledged and spoken into, it often loses its power.

The opposite pole of fear is faith. I suggest that a regular relaxation or prayer practice can acknowledge fear without being caught in its power.

Endometriosis

Endometriosis is fairly common; twelve million women have the diagnosis in the United States. The exact cause isn't known, although one theory is that when the lining of the uterus flows out during menstruation, some of the cells are moved "backwards" up and out the tubes to fall into the abdominal cavity. These cells then implant in the pelvis and "cycle" just as the endometrium or lining of the uterus cycles. When the implanted cells cycle, it can make scars and weblike connections between the organs called *adhesions*. The implanted cells are called endometriosis; they can be on the surface of the uterus, the tubes, the ovaries, the bowels and the bladder. They can even travel to other parts of the body such as the lungs. The most common symptoms of endometriosis are pain with menstruation, pain with intercourse and pain with a bowel movement.

Although pelvic examinations and ultrasounds can sometimes show the suggestion of endometriosis, the only sure way to diagnose this disease is to look inside the abdomen. This is usually done with a laparoscope. A laparoscope is a surgical instrument with a camera attached that can fit through a small incision in the belly button. Gynecologists are trained to recognize and treat the endometriosis using the laparoscope; the surgery is usually done as an outpatient with general anesthesia.

Other traditional approaches to endometriosis include the use of hormones to decrease the pain. Rather than review which hormones are used here, I'm going to suggest that you discuss this with your gynecologist and decide if this is the right approach for you.

Severe pain warrants surgery or evaluation, so I'm going to review some integrative therapies and techniques that are appropriate for milder symptoms. I caution everyone to follow their symptoms closely and to have them evaluated if they don't improve with these suggestions.

Nutrition is, again, my first and possibly most important treatment suggestion. Endometriosis can be worsened by estrogen dominance. We are exposed in our environment to many chemicals that act on our body like estrogen. Pesticides and other chemicals are hard to avoid; remember to wash all fruits and vegetables before eating them. Try to buy organic products whenever possible. Pay special attention to cruciferous vegetables such as broccoli, cauliflower, cabbage and Brussels sprouts along with soy and essential fatty acids such as fish oil to help your body break down estrogen more efficiently and safely.

Relaxation and visualization daily can help reframe your "wiring" and make a difference in pain perception. My patients have had good results with castor oil packs on the abdomen (cloth soaked with castor oil in a plastic casing with a heating pad on top). While the warm pack is in place, visualize balance and perfect order. Turn off the television and the radio. Turn off the computer. Unplug the phone. In our busy, over-scheduled lives, it takes conviction and commitment to slow down and "stop"—if only for an hour or so.

A gentle pelvic massage with warmed oil can also help the pelvic muscles relax and ease the pain. As you may recall from our discussion of fibroids, the pelvis is the energy center for creativity and connection. Focus on where the disconnect is in your life. Listen for the messages your body is sending you. Journal with open-ended statements as your starting point. Examples could be these: "the way I feel about my life is …" or "the way I feel about my job is …" or "the way I feel about my relationship is …" Journaling is something that gets easier with time; commit to fifteen minutes a day and see if the discipline makes a difference.

Acupuncture has been shown to decrease pain from endometriosis (although this ancient technique was developed before the disease was recognized pathologically). Fine needles are inserted in the arms, legs and abdomen to balance the energy. While the needles are in place, relax and settle into a peaceful, pain-free energetic balance.

Pelvic physical therapy can also help with pelvic pain. Since pain causes muscle tension (or perhaps muscle tension causes pelvic pain), a skilled therapist can train you to relax and strengthen the various muscles of the pelvis. Not all physical therapists specialize in treating the pelvis—ask your gynecologist for a referral to one who does.

Integrating nutrition, relaxation, journaling and pelvic physical therapy can make the diagnosis of endometriosis less dire, but best of all it can make a difference in the intensity of pelvic pain and the quality of life.

5

Fertility

A Burst of Life—Preparing the Soil

"I hate birth announcements," a patient told me recently. "It's not that I'm not happy for my friends that are having kids, it's just that every time I get one in the mail it brings up this wash of feelings—feelings of sadness, frustration and anger because I'm not pregnant."

It's the essence of who we are—and yet there aren't many discussions that can bring up a more heated debate and a wider range of emotions than reproduction.

Our ability to reproduce is an intricate dance of timing, hormonal support and physical potential. The dance involves a man and a woman with their individual, unique anatomy and physiology. The resulting pregnancy combines genetic information from both parents, and the cycle continues from generation to generation again and again. There are varying rates of success with fertility; a couple is considered "subfertile" if they don't achieve pregnancy within a year of regular intercourse without contraception.

I'll discuss pregnancy itself later in this book, but if pregnancy *doesn't* just occur, there are as many reasons why as there are couples looking for the answer. Simplistically, pregnancy requires an egg, a sperm, an open fallopian tube and a uterus that can implant and support the new pregnancy for nine months. What we know is that 40 percent of the time the fertility problem involves either releasing an egg (ovulation) or problems with tubes or uterine structure; 40 percent of the time it is a problem with the number and/or quality of sperm; and 20 percent of the time we don't know why there's a problem!

A woman usually starts the fertility evaluation with her gynecologist who reviews her menstrual cycles, her medical history, her current medications and vitamins. She is started on a prenatal vitamin, ideally before conception. Her gynecologist will also ask about her use of tobacco, alcohol and other drugs. A physical exam with a Pap smear and infection screening is then followed with checking and updating her immunizations including German measles or rubella and varicella or chicken pox. If she works around body fluids, the hepatitis B vaccine is given along with a tuberculosis screen. Other possible immunizations include the flu shot and an updated tetanus vaccination. In addition, women in northern latitudes should consider screening their vitamin D levels, which may be too low.

Measuring *basal body temperatures* is an inexpensive way to see if and when ovulation occurs. Look up this phrase in your favorite Internet search engine, and you'll be led to sites that will chart your temperatures for you and help predict the day of egg release. Your job, then, is to "hook up" with your husband on the appropriate day and complete the act of co-creation.

If pregnancy *still* doesn't occur, the next step is usually seeing a reproductive endocrinologist, a board-certified ob-gyn who has completed a fellowship that includes advanced training in surgical and medical treatments of fertility. The work-up continues, and strategies for achieving pregnancy are mapped out.

I have patients who approach their fertility as if it were one more examination to study for or one more achievement to work toward. They've been successful in so many areas of their lives— this one area frustrates them.

The problem with this approach to pregnancy is that it can lead to a mindset that focuses on the mechanical process and timing of reproduction. As you can imagine, a loving relationship can become strained as lovemaking becomes timed and "required" rather than spontaneous and voluntary. In addition, an internal "war" is set up as menstrual cycles are dreaded and resented, ticking off time and reproductive potential.

I'd like to reframe this discussion and put it in the context of Imbolc, one of the four principal festivals of the Irish calendar, also known St. Brigid's Day. Imbolc (*Imbolg* or "in the belly" referring to the pregnancy and lactation of ewes) is midway between the winter solstice and the spring equinox, typically celebrated on the first of February. This is the celebration of the beginnings of spring, and it is the time to ready the ground for planting. Correlate that concept with a uterus; it needs to be in balance and ready for implantation of the new pregnancy. So what can you do to assist this balance?

Look at your job and your life balance. Are you happy? Are you stimulated and nurtured? Now is the time to nurture your body with healthy, nutritious food. Adding at least 400 micrograms of folic acid (a B vitamin) can decrease the incidence of some birth defects. In addition to fruits and vegetables and folic acid, it's time to exercise and stretch and dance and laugh. It's time to nurture your relationship with time and energy. Journal a list of the things you love and cherish about your partner. Remember why you fell in love and what you want in your lives as you live and grow together.

Slow down and look at that crocus that just broke through the ground. The "burst of life" after the frost and snow reminds us that the cycle of life is miraculous and powerful. Look at the beauty around you—maybe the ice on the branches is delicate and lacy, maybe the sky showed you more shades of blue and gray than you've ever seen before. Look around and *really see* the beauty!

Integrative Fertility Baby Steps

Most of us understand that the steps needed in fertility are (1) the preparation and release of an egg, (2) the fertilization of the egg with a sperm, followed by (3) the implantation of the fertilized egg in the uterus where it grows and develops into a baby. Each of these steps is intricate and complex.

Fertility specialists have developed increasingly elaborate medications and procedures to assist couples with these "baby steps." Yet despite all the interventions and studies, fully 20 to 30 percent of couples have "unexplained" infertility. Several studies have evaluated the addition of less traditional and more integrative therapies for fertility. I suggest we use the following therapies *alongside of or in combination with* rather than as an *alternative* to traditional medicine's fertility treatments.

- **Acupuncture**: The integrative therapy that has the most supportive data for infertility is acupuncture. Acupuncture uses fine sterile needles in the body in patterns that are designed to assist with fertility.

Studies have shown that acupuncture can increase the number of times that a woman ovulates. (For women with irregular cycles or PCOS (polycystic ovarian syndrome), this therapy can be very helpful.) In a similar way, acupuncture can help increase the number and quality of sperm that a man produces.

Acupuncture has also been used to decrease the pain during egg retrieval during an IVF (in vitro fertilization) cycle. Perhaps most exciting to women and their caregivers is the increase in pregnancy rates when acupuncture is used in IVF cycles. Over a dozen studies have now been done where women are treated similarly but half are given acupuncture treatments during their IVF cycles. Again and again there is an increase in the pregnancy rates in the acupuncture-treated patients.

- **Chiropractic:** Adjustments, especially of the lumbar spine, may also help with the pregnancy "baby steps." Because the nerves and blood vessels of the pelvis travel through and around the spine, doctors of chiropractic medicine believe that adjusting the spine can improve blood flow and hormonal communication in fertility patients. There have been fewer randomized controlled trials in this area, but I can report from my practice that we've seen a nice result when chiropractic adjustments are included in the fertility plan.

- **Massage therapy:** Massage therapy can improve fertility rates in a few different ways. Relaxation helps to lower the stress hormone cortisol. The hormonal symphony of fertility is more paced and harmonic. The busy, over-booked, exhausted woman who is trying to conceive a pregnancy has to stop, relax and rebalance. Some licensed massage therapists are trained to do a uterine massage that is designed to improve blood flow to the pelvis for ovulation and implantation. Again there are no randomized controlled trials, but I have seen many success stories.

- **Craniosacral therapy:** Similar to massage, craniosacral therapy can improve fertility rates by both relaxation and improved hormonal balance. Craniosacral therapists apply gentle pressure to the skull bones and the vertebral column including the sacral bone in the pelvis to create "waves" of cerebrospinal fluid through the body. The treatment is relaxing and extremely helpful for clients with neck pain, migraines and other muscle pains.

- **Energy therapies:** Energy therapies such as healing touch or Reiki treatments can also be an important part of fertility care. Practitioners use gentle touch and intuition to work within the individual's energy body to regain optimal balance and relaxation. Deep relaxation is a "side effect" of energy therapy. Again randomized trials are lacking.

Integrative therapies can improve fertility success for couples trying to take "baby steps" toward starting a family. Relaxation and less pain are the most common side effects of integrative therapies. Reimbursements for most fertility treatments are spotty and employer-dependent.

I encourage couples to start with the basics—a good healthy nutritious diet of colorful fruits and vegetables, a vitamin supplement that includes at least 400 micrograms of folic acid and at least 1 gram of fish oil (EPA and DHA) or another omega-3 fatty acid. In addition to nutrition, I encourage a small amount of light exercise daily such as walking or yoga. I also ask couples to include a daily meditative quiet time to force them to slow down and unwind from the day's tensions and stresses. Together we explore the particular integrative therapies available and design a program that fits with their needs and budget.

Integrative Treatments for Pregnancy

An oak tree exists within the cellular framework of an acorn. Given the correct conditions and time, a sunflower seed has the capacity to develop into a tall beautiful sunflower. A human sperm fertilizes a human egg and the two cells become millions. Within our mother's womb, our bodies took form and shape and organized into layers of cells that became muscles and clumps of cells that became organs. Human pregnancy and childbirth almost always proceeds as if it were on "cruise control." In other words, we have no conscious awareness of fetal development other than the physical discomforts that occur as the child grows and the uterus expands in size.

An integrative approach to pregnancy starts with the awareness of co-creation. Chinese medicine describes the formation of life as "form from nothingness." The ancient texts describe fetal development as a "transition from anterior heaven to posterior heaven" that allows an "energetic ordering" to matter. As with the oak tree or sunflower, the developing fetus requires nourishing energy, moisture and time. Nourishing energy should come in the form of regular relaxation breathing/meditation and a whole food diet with a focus on colorful organic vegetables and fruit. Pregnant mothers should supplement with at least 2 grams of high-quality EPA/DHA (fish oil) and insure they take a high-quality prenatal vitamin with at least 400 micrograms of folic acid daily—both preferably *before* conception. In addition, as I mentioned before, women in northern latitudes should consider screening their vitamin D levels and supplementing as needed.

Complaints of nausea in the first trimester are seen as an interruption in the normal "flow" of life force energy in the pregnant mother. Eastern medicine describes this as "rebellious qi" (pronounced *chee* or *kee*), and acupuncture and other energetic treatments can balance and alleviate the symptoms. The acupuncture needles are placed on the arms, legs, stomach and sometimes ear of the pregnant woman. One point that can be used with pressure alone is the underside of the wrist between the tendons (elastic bands called "Sea bands" with a bead are sometimes used for nausea—placing the bead in this point). Other strategies to use for nausea during pregnancy include changing your eating patterns to the practice of consuming small, frequent meals and avoiding strongly flavored or spicy foods.

Ginger can be used to calm the stomach—grate a ginger root and then steep it with hot water, strain the liquid and use a small amount of honey or stevia for sweetening. Sip it slowly when it is warm or cold; be consciously aware of your feet and legs and your connection to the earth. Perhaps play a guided imagery affirmation or other relaxing music during this time. You are consciously connecting to the power of co-creation while affirming your groundedness and strength.

Another pregnancy complaint is low back pain and hip pain as the pregnant uterus grows larger in the last trimester of gestation. Pregnancy support belts can help with the abdominal pressure and discomfort; chiropractic adjustments and massage are important tools to use as needed. Acupuncture can work in conjunction with the chiropractic care to relieve muscle tension and pain. The key to muscle discomfort in pregnancy is posture, stretching and core strengthening.

Find a prenatal yoga class that helps you in all of these areas and practice the stretches daily. After almost twenty years of delivering babies, I can tell you that my patients who were actively stretching and exercising during their pregnancies had fewer aches and pains during the final weeks of pregnancy and had more stamina overall when labor started.

Exceptions to the rule when it comes to exercise include pregnancies with more than one developing fetus and those at high risk for preterm labor. Ask your physician or midwife about exercise limits and listen to your body. Any symptom such as spotting, low abdominal pain or pressure or a persistent vaginal discharge should be reported and evaluated. Premature labor and delivery is a huge cause of infant mortality; don't take a chance here! The March of Dimes has an excellent Web site that reviews warning signs and symptoms at www.marchofdimes.com.

The last area I'll mention to those of you who are currently pregnant or are planning a pregnancy soon is in the area of emotional preparedness for parenting. The least helpful statement I heard during my pregnancy almost twenty years ago was, "It'll change your life!" said with an overtone of warning. I know that choosing pregnancy and parenting takes commitment and courage. Connect to the best that is within you and your partner. If necessary, explore your own childhood experience with a mental health professional and release patterns that no longer serve you. Recognize that as parents we do our best to nurture and guide the next generation as best we can.

The Business of Being Born—At Home!

This section is going to verge on the political. And maybe it won't have a lot of integrative medicine in it. And maybe it will discuss issues that you hadn't thought about or been exposed to before. And maybe it will push a couple of buttons here or there. Let me explain.

In November 2007 I served on a panel leading a discussion after the local screening of *The Business of Being Born*, a film directed by Sara Epstein and produced by Ricki Lake, the actress and former talk-show host. The film's screening in my town was a fundraiser for the local chapter of the International Cesarean Awareness Network (ICAN). I was joined on the panel by a lactation consultant, two nurse midwives and a direct-entry midwife. More on the movie later.

Let's talk about midwives first. A nurse midwife (CNM) is a registered nurse (RN) who has done the equivalent of a master's degree in midwifery and is qualified to provide primary care for women including gynecologic care as well as prenatal, labor, delivery and postpartum care. In Ohio where I practice, CNMs are certified through the Ohio Board of Nursing. Each state has its own certification criteria (similar to physicians who are licensed separately by each state in which they practice). In Cincinnati where I live, there are currently about two dozen practicing nurse midwives, and there is an active training program at the University of Cincinnati School of Nursing. CNMs deliver babies at all of the area hospitals in Cincinnati and have ob-gyn physicians as back-up in case a surgical delivery (forceps or cesarean section) is necessary. There are no longer any CNMs who provide home births in Cincinnati, and the only birth center in town closed in 2007. This happened because of pressure from malpractice carriers to their back-up physicians even though statistics show that midwife-attended births are less likely to result in a malpractice suit.

Direct-entry midwives or Certified Professional Midwives (CPM) are trained specifically in prenatal care, newborn care and home births through accredited training programs and home birth experience. They practice legally in thirty-four states and are certified in twenty states. (Ohio is not a state where CPMs practice or are certified.) After much study, a bill was introduced in 2002 (Ohio HB477), which would have set up a Midwifery Board to regulate and license these midwives. The bill had widespread support from the home birth community, but it remained in committee and expired that year. At this point, a woman who wants to have a home birth has few (if any) options in Cincinnati. Which brings me back to the movie and its agenda.

The movie was released nationally in January 2008 and follows several direct-entry midwives through the preparation and deliveries of several home births. Intermixed with the home birth sequences is a history of obstetrics in our country including a shot of an active hospital's labor and delivery board with "pitocin" (a drug used to induce and augment labor) and "epidural" (a type of anesthesia) next to almost every patient's name.

According to the Agency for Healthcare Research and Quality, we spend $7,600 per uncomplicated pregnancy in the United States. We spend more than most developed countries on prenatal care and have a higher infant mortality rate. (We're number twenty-five in the world.) The movie is quite clear in its implication that intervention in the normal process of labor and birth impacts bonding between a mother and her child. In addition, the movie wonders out loud if each technological advance in obstetrical care such as the routine use of continuous fetal monitoring has really been a step forward for low-risk women and their babies.

I don't question the movie's passion and verve. The final birth in the movie is of Sara Epstein's own labor and delivery four weeks before her due date. She was assessed by her CPM at her home and immediately transported to the hospital because her baby was still breech (not presenting head first). The back-up obstetrician delivered her son by cesarean section, and he is doing well today, according to the movie's Web site.

So what's the issue? Do I want to have a home birth? Well the short answer is no. After delivering thousands of babies, I can assure you that the hours of waiting followed by moments of hyper-alert awareness resulted in many births that would have been absolutely appropriate and safe at home. There were a few births, though, when I was grateful to have the ability to instantly deliver or resuscitate a baby. *But that is my training and my perspective.* I've never attended a home birth. I wasn't trained to evaluate who was appropriate for home birth and who needed to be transported. I did see hundreds of un-medicated labors and births though. I can tell you that it is tremendously powerful to watch a laboring woman who chooses to walk and move and moan with the power of her contractions. Her strength and resolve are awe-inspiring. The final "darkness before dawn" is a challenge for everyone in the delivery room. The postscript of the alert, quiet, nursing child and the proud warrior/survivor mom can still bring tears of joy to my eyes.

This movie brought me to tears several times. Birth can do that—as a baby makes a safe transition between the world of maternal support to independent life. What it didn't do was talk about the *business* of being born, such as the community expectation that every birth will result in a healthy, perfect baby, or the beliefs that if something is wrong with the baby then *someone* must be at fault. Perhaps a blip on the monitor was missed or an intervention wasn't done in time. The ever-present lawyers, malpractice companies and the national practitioner database where all of us who practice obstetrics have at least one notation by our names. The insurance companies. The professional societies. The medical instrumentation companies. That business of being born ... now *that* would be quite a movie.

Breastfeeding and Breast Health

October is breast cancer awareness month. During the month, you're likely to see a pink ribbon somewhere. On clothing. On pens. On mugs. Like the yellow ribbons for returning soldiers and the red ribbons for AIDS awareness, the pink ribbons are designed to make us aware of the incidence of breast cancer in our country and encourage research toward a cure.

Most people are aware that one in eight women in the United States in her lifetime will develop breast cancer. The CDC's Web site notes that 186,772 women and 1,815 men were diagnosed with breast cancer in 2004 (the most recent year for which numbers are available). Breast cancer is number six of the top ten causes of death for women (heart disease is the runaway number one killer of women), and, like many health-related issues in our country, there is a racial disparity in treatment success. Caucasian women have the highest incidence of breast cancer; however, black women are more likely to die of the disease. Also, interestingly enough, after a slow but steady increase in the incidence of breast cancer through the last few decades, there has been a statistically significant decrease in both incidence and death from breast cancer from 2001 to 2004.

But rather than talk about cancer and death, what I'd really rather get you excited about is breast health—optimal physical, emotional, mental and spiritual health where your breasts are concerned. What does that sound like to you? There is an odd cultural attitude toward women's breasts in our country. We've turned a functional, nurturing part of our anatomy into a sexual focus. There's a cultural expectation that we should undergo enlargement with implants if our breast size is too small and reduction with surgery if our breast size is too big. And because our breasts are situated anatomically right over our heart, they are a magnifying focus for negative emotional energy from heartbreak and loss.

Anatomically, our breasts are fairly straightforward. There's a web of connective tissue with blood vessels surrounding a network of glands. Body fat "fills in the gaps" and provides the contour and texture. The fat also serves as a "storage silo" for hormones and their metabolites. Breasts serve the amazing function of milk production for our newborn child after birth. There is an elaborate dance of hormones that interweaves after labor and suckling. A relaxed, unstressed and nourished new mother produces milk easily and bountifully for her relaxed and unstressed child. Nature allows a smaller volume, higher protein colostrum to serve as nourishment and "immune system booster" until regular breast milk is created within a few days after birth.

Before and after pregnancies and breastfeeding, our breasts respond to our menstrual cycle hormones by increasing in size and gland complexity. We learn quickly that the hormonal fluctuations in our cycles can result in full, tender breasts if we are out of balance from a nutrition or stress standpoint.

What has become clear in the last five to ten years is that we each have a unique genetic signature that describes how we remove female hormones from our body. It's clear that some of the pathways of metabolism result in metabolites that are safer and less likely to cause DNA damage and cancer in our cells while some pathways are less safe. Not only can we measure this genetic "fingerprint" of metabolic pathways, but we can also measure the products of metabolism and watch them change as we change our diet and nutritional supplementation. Products such as high-quality fish oil, antioxidants and cruciferous vegetables can basically decrease the "flow" down the bad metabolic pathway and shunt toward the safer one. What's more, we have a tool to use if we choose to take hormone replacement during or after menopause to guide us in the selection of which type of hormone to use.

Not only can we clear toxins and toxic metabolites from our breast tissues, but we can also learn how to clear toxic emotions from our body and spirit. Emotional, mental and physical abuse can leave unseen scars on our mind, body (heart and breasts) and spirit. We can tap into networks and therapists and religious ministries that help us process the abuse and clear it from our system.

Steve Sherwood, a facilitator at Life Success Seminars in Cincinnati (www.lifesuccessseminars.com) uses the phrase "shards of glass"—as though a picture "shattered" and caused pain that is still lodged in our hearts. He describes ways of releasing and removing those shards. Not surprisingly, perhaps, the answer is love, gratitude and reaching for our dreams and releasing our past. Along the way we learn to trust, forgive and focus on making responsible choices in our lives.

I hope these thoughts give you pause to stop and appreciate your breasts. Now let's celebrate and keep them healthy!

The Ins and Outs of Contraception

I've recognized the controversy around contraception since my early medical school days. My classmates and I all received free materials from a local organization that had a strong opinion about contraception and family planning services. As my practice experience continued, I learned how to ask questions so that I could learn at the office visit if contraceptive advice was desired without offending a woman who felt contraception was not in line with her religious beliefs.

For a few years, I joined the Couple to Couple League, an organization that teaches natural family planning, so that I had an idea how to counsel and advise my patients who used this method. These patients followed their basal body temperatures, cervical mucus and menstrual cycles carefully and accurately and chose the timing of their children's births. This section is not written to them or for them. This discussion is written for the women of reproductive age who are interested in delaying or avoiding pregnancy and do not have the time or support from their partner to practice natural family planning.

The Guttmacher Institute notes that the typical American woman wants only two children. To achieve this goal, she must use a contraceptive method for roughly three decades. The Institute also reports that among the forty-two million fertile, heterosexual, sexually active women who do not want to become pregnant, 89 percent use contraception of some type. The type of contraception is generally age-specific. Younger women mostly use condoms or birth control pills, while women over thirty-five years of age are more likely to use female sterilization.

Women have an array of methods for preventing pregnancy. Barrier methods such as male condoms are widely available and relatively inexpensive. Their first-year contraceptive failure rate can vary from 2 percent in a "perfect user" to 17.4 percent in a "typical user." Condoms can decrease (although not eliminate) the spread of sexually transmitted infections. They are relatively easy to use with rare side effects. A female condom has been on the market for a few decades; its cost ($4) is roughly four times the price of a male condom.

The FDA first approved the birth control pill in the 1960s. The formulation and strength of synthetic estrogens and progestins have varied from pill to pill. The first-year contraceptive failure rate for the pill varies from 0.3 percent for a perfect user to 8.7 percent for an average user. The pill works by mimicking the hormonal fluctuations of a normal menstrual cycle. Ovulation rates decrease (and subsequently pregnancy rates). Noncontraceptive benefits of the pill have also been shown. The lifetime risk of ovarian cancer is decreased in women who have used the pill for at least three months. Menstrual cycles are lighter and with less intense cramping. The pill can effectively treat acne and other skin conditions.

There are downsides to the pill. There is an increased risk of blood clots and stroke. The pill is less effective in women with a BMI over 27 (equivalent to a 5-foot-4-inch tall woman weighing 160 pounds or more). In addition, the lower dose pills almost require a regular routine of pill taking. Missing a pill, taking it late or taking a medication such as an antibiotic that increases the rate of hormone metabolism by the liver will lower hormone levels and lead to spotting and/or an unplanned pregnancy.

Because of the inconvenience of daily pill consumption, drug manufacturers have offered three-month injections, five-year implants (no longer on the market), vaginal rings, and patches (no longer on the market). There is also a formulation that skips the "monthly" cycles and changes the bleeding pattern to quarterly. (Their marketing equates menstrual cycles as something to be endured, while the pharmaceutical company plays the part of the white knight rescuing the damsel in distress. I abhor this attitude toward women and their menstrual cycles. If you missed the section on menstruation, go back and read it!)

Intrauterine devices (IUDs) are designed to prevent pregnancy by both preventing fertilization (changing cervical mucus to prevent sperm penetration) and preventing implantation of a newly fertilized egg. The history of implanting a foreign object in the womb to prevent pregnancy is ancient and multicultural. There are currently two types of IUDs available. Most women who choose the IUD like the convenience and have had at least one child. The disadvantages of the method are the risk of infection and potential sterility. One IUD, the Dalkon shield, was taken off the market in 1974 after the risk of pelvic inflammatory disease was found to be five times higher than other IUDs on the market.

Are contraceptive options uniformly safe, easy to use and available to all women and their partners who wish to use them? The short answer is no. We know that women's and children's health are both improved when contraception is available to space pregnancies and assist in the prevention of sexually transmitted infections. We also know that the worldwide access to contraception and family planning is closely tied to promoting economic growth and social stability. Again, quoting the Guttmacher Institute

"Families that can choose the number, timing and spacing of their children are better able to plan their lives, to save resources and to increase their household income. Families with more children have a higher risk of falling into poverty. Having fewer children allows parents to invest in their existing children and provide adequate nutrition, housing and education for the entire family. Moreover, women who control their fertility have more time for their own development and are more able to socially and politically participate in their communities."

Pap Smears and the HPV Vaccine

George Papanicolaou rocked the gynecology world in the 1940s by introducing an effective screening tool for cervical cancer. We continue to honor his accomplishment by calling the screening method a "Pap smear" although our methods have evolved since his day. The strategy, then and now, is to sample and detect cells that are in the process of changing to cancer before they become invasive.

According to the National Cancer Institute, the incidence of cervical cancer decreased by 43 percent from 1973 and 1995. Cervical cancer was once the *leading cause* of cancer death in women in the 1950s; it has now dropped to below the top ten. No one doubts that we have an effective tool to screen for this type of cancer. But the problems are these: (1) the Pap smear requires a speculum and a somewhat uncomfortable exam; and (2) we have unequal access to health care throughout our country and the world. So let's face it, a screening tool is only effective if it is used!

We know that there were about 11,000 new cases of cervical cancer diagnosed in 2008 in the United States and that 4,000 women will die from the disease in one year. We also now know that cervical cancer is caused by exposure to and infection by the human papillomavirus (HPV). HPV is the most common sexually transmitted infection in the United States. Some studies suggest that 80 percent of us will be exposed to the virus by the time we are fifty. Most young women who are exposed to the virus "clear" it from their systems within two to three years. (You might wonder why I don't have data on young men and their infection rates? Ah, well, welcome to the separate and not-quite-equal world of health care!) Factors that cause the virus to persist include a genetic predisposition, a suppressed immune system and cigarette smoking. There are over a hundred different types or strains of HPV; we classify some of the types as "high risk" strains—or the ones most likely to cause cancer. The virus is passed by direct contact with the skin—one reason why condoms don't completely prevent its transmission.

With this background, drug companies stepped up research to develop a vaccine for HPV, and Merck won FDA approval for its vaccine Guardisil in June 2006. The vaccine contains non-infectious virus particles and is designed to prevent the infection of HPV types 16 and 18 (which cause 70 percent of cervical cancers) and HPV types 6 and 11 (which cause 90 percent of genital warts). There was a tremendous lobbying effort to approve the vaccine.

At the time of the approval, fewer than 12,000 girls had been studied with follow-up for five years or more. Although there are data on vaccine efficacy for girls ages nine to twenty-five, the biggest trial data are on sixteen to twenty-five-year-olds. The CDC and the Advisory Committee on Immunization Practices (ACIP) recommends routine vaccination of girls aged eleven to twelve.

Some states are wrestling with the thorny issue of whether the HPV vaccine should be mandatory for all girls. Obviously, the goal of the age recommendation is to vaccinate before the girls become sexually active. Three doses of the vaccine are given over the course of six months; the cost now is $125 per dose. It makes sense mathematically that if the majority of girls are vaccinated, then the incidence of cervical cancer will decrease by at least 70 percent in the next two decades.

So let's be clear here. This is a vaccine that's designed to prevent cancer and genital warts. It doesn't prevent all sexually transmitted infections (abstinence is the only sure-fire way to completely prevent them), and it doesn't mean we can be complacent and decrease or stop cervical cancer (Pap smear) screening. There is also no reason to assume that vaccinating our daughters will increase sexual promiscuity. (One public health researcher likened this argument to assuming that seat belts in a car caused reckless driving.)

What the vaccine does is prevent infection for these four types of HPV for at least five years. Merck is continuing to monitor the immunity status; we'll know more as time unfolds. The company's ads that say, "One less!" should have an asterisk that says, "For at least five years for 70 percent of cancers and 90 percent of genital warts." As parents, we need to evaluate our comfort level with using a vaccine that is relatively new.

We also need to continue to keep the lines of communication open where sexuality is concerned. Remember those teen years?

When we were teens, we grew up physically long before we grew up mentally and emotionally. As teens we're learning what it means to be a woman, a friend, a lover. As parents of a teen, we might find that a loving, rational, fact-based discussion of relationships, life stressors and choices is the best vaccine of all!

6

Menopause

Aging Gracefully

The great thing about getting older is that you don't lose all the other ages you've been.

Madeline L'Engle

We've all seen the stories of the aging baby boomers and the graying of America. Most people know that the increased birth rate after World War II resulted in a peak of births roughly fifty years ago. Government data state that 12 percent of the population is currently over sixty-five. In thirty years, this number will be more than 20 percent. In addition, because our life expectancy has lengthened to the early eighties, most of us will spend a third of our lives after our last menstrual cycle.

The average age of menopause is fifty-one, which by definition means no menstrual cycle for a year. The time frame five to ten years prior to menopause is called the perimenopause or climacteric. Most symptoms associated with menopause begin during the perimenopausal period. Hot flashes, changes in sleep patterns, mood changes (especially anger or depression), libido changes and weight gain are the most common complaints that I hear. (I'll review symptoms and treatments later in this chapter, by the way.) Interestingly enough, menopausal symptoms are different for every woman and the suggestions about coping with symptoms are just as varied. In addition to the symptomatic complaints, I find that a woman in this age range is often brought face to face with her own fears about aging and her own mortality.

Some women and their physicians choose to add hormones to help decrease their symptoms for a few years during the perimenopausal transition. At this moment the hormonal discussion in our country is occurring on many levels including the government, the ob-gyn establishment, the drug companies, the practitioners and the pharmacies, to name just a few. It's apparent that women (and some practitioners) are confused about hormonal options. Best-selling authors have brought this discussion into the mainstream; I'll step into the swirl of controversy and discuss hormone therapy shortly.

But first, why does menopause occur? The simple medical answer is that our ovaries gradually stop producing the hormones estrogen and progesterone. Without the signaling, the lining of the uterus or endometrium stops building up and sloughing. But why does this occur? Why not cycle our hormones indefinitely? There have been theories and suggestions, but the real answer isn't known. Regardless of the reason, it appears we were designed to start cycling in puberty and stop in our fourth or fifth decade. Earlier, I discussed the web of hormones that allows the menstrual cycle to take place—the hormonal symphony—the series of hormonal cues. In menopause the same hormonal symphony is gradually changing and winding down.

In my role as a physician, my job is to make sure that the menstrual cycle changes aren't because of an anatomic problem with the uterus or ovaries or a problem with one of the other hormones such as thyroid or adrenal. In addition, menopause is an excellent platform to discuss health in general and encourage health screenings such as Pap smears, mammograms, blood work, colonoscopies and bone density screenings. Lifestyle habits such as regular exercise, healthy nutrition and regular meditation or prayer can be reviewed and encouraged.

Aging gracefully is not an accident. We bring our genetic predisposition to age-related illnesses such as heart disease or arthritis, but our future is not rigidly set. We can bathe our genes in the environmental cues of nutritious and colorful organic fruits and vegetables. We can move our bodies and stretch each day. We can acknowledge our life stressors and continue to work toward life balance and resilience. Our attitude and our outlook pave the way for healthy life choices. We can surround ourselves with people who support us in our choices. We can practice laughing.

Nonhormonal Treatments for Common Menopausal Symptoms

In this section I'll begin a review of the symptoms of menopause and discuss an integrative approach to embracing them. I believe it's important to acknowledge our menopausal symptoms as flash points (pun intended!) for awareness about our body and our menopausal transition.

Hot Flashes

Hot flashes are by far the most common complaint I hear from perimenopausal women. They are usually experienced as a rush of heat from the center of the body up to the head and can be associated with sweating, an increase in the heart rate and varying degrees of anxiety. (By the way, the experience of hot flashes varies from woman to woman and culture to culture—some women have few if any hot flashes. Remember that as a gynecologist, I'm more likely to see women with symptoms in my office so my experience is slightly skewed.)

The exact cause of hot flashes isn't known. We know that the triggers can be hormonal fluctuation, spicy food or emotional stimuli, among others, but the exact physiology of the hot flash is rooted in the hypothalamus at the base of the brain. Within the hypothalamus is our body's "thermostat" that allows shivering with cold air and sweating with hot air. Apparently the thermostat loses its tight control on temperature regulation.

Christiane Northrup, MD, describes this period of a woman's life as a time of "re-wiring"—as if our cells are changing from the cyclic hormonal fluctuations of our reproductive years to a steady-state postmenopausal pattern.

Regardless of the reason for the hot flashes, several integrative approaches can be taken to decrease them.

- Breathe: My first recommendation is to breathe. Just breathe. Researchers have shown that paced breathing can decrease the severity and frequency of hot flashes by 50 to 60 percent. With the onset of a hot flash, try to sit or stand with your feet flat on the floor and become aware of the bottoms of your feet. Breathe in slowly for a count of three, hold your breath for a count of three and breathe out slowly for a count of three. This gets easier with practice. Imagine that the bottoms of your feet are tapped into an unlimited "power source" of innate goodness or grace. Bring that power up into your lungs and heart and expel any anger, fear or sadness right back down into that source. Repeat this exercise for a few minutes whenever necessary.

- Acupuncture: Another effective treatment for hot flashes is acupuncture. In Chinese medicine, a hot flash is an energetic imbalance that can be treated with acupuncture needles and herbs. Energetic balance is typically achieved after two to three months of weekly or biweekly treatments. Acupuncture uses fine sterile needles in the arms, legs and body to achieve this balance. A common "side-effect" of acupuncture is a sense of relaxation and peace. In this day of overbooked lives I like to encourage women to slow down and stop—if only for thirty minutes or so on my treatment table.

- Energy medicine: An adjunct to energetic balance for hot flashes is energy medicine such as Reiki or healing touch. Practitioners who are trained in energy medicine use their hands to move and balance energy in their clients. I find that the combination of acupuncture needles and the hands of an energy medicine practitioner is an ideal treatment for my clients with severe hot flashes.

- Nutrition and nutritional supplements: These approaches can also be used to treat hot flashes. Some foods are more likely to interfere with hormonal balance (white sugar, white flour, trans fats), while some foods are more likely to achieve hormonal balance and optimal hormonal metabolism (broccoli and Brussels sprouts to name just a few). High-quality supplements with isoflavones and phytoestrogens from plants such as black cohosh, kudzu and red clover can be helpful. Geranium oil applied directly to your wrists, knees and behind your ears can also help hot flashes. My rule of thumb for supplements is *one bottle as directed*. If you haven't seen a change in symptoms after one bottle, stop and ask for advice. Because supplements are not regulated in this country, I suggest using products that follow good manufacturing procedures and do "batch testing" for the active ingredients. I also suggest that you bring in the bottle of any supplement you're taking when you see your health practitioner. If they look at you cross-eyed or discount your questions, get another opinion.

Above all, don't look for the solution to your hot flashes in a pill. Look at the big picture. Look at your life balance and your nutrition. And don't forget to breathe!

Libido and Sexuality

Decreased libido or sexual desire is a frequent complaint of menopausal and perimenopausal women. As always, before we review treatments, let's review what we know about sexuality and libido.

Sexuality is part of our individual health and wholeness. Besides being the basis for reproduction and the survival of our species, it adds a dimension to the communication between two people in a committed relationship. For the purpose of this discussion I'm going to talk about heterosexuality, although some if not most of this discussion will translate to lesbian relationships.

To start with, libido is an emotional and mental desire for sexual intimacy. Our attitudes toward our sexual health start early. We observe affection (or its lack!) in our family of origin; we stumble into adolescence and experiment with our feelings and our bodies. Our culture and our religions have specific expectations and rules of behavior both in and around sexual relationships. These rules vary between families and religions, but in general we are ultimately drawn to a committed monogamous union. Two adults in a committed relationship can often run into difficulties when their physical bodies age and change as they do in menopause (and andropause for men).

The most common physical change of menopause that affects sexuality is vaginal dryness or decreased lubrication. This can lead to discomfort and pain with intercourse and sometimes an increased incidence in vaginal and bladder infections. Understandably, if sex hurts, libido is affected. If vaginal dryness is the complaint, I'd suggest a pelvic exam by a gynecology practitioner to confirm that there are no infections or other physical reasons for the pain or dryness.

If everything checks out, then explore the pace and the timing of your sexual relationship. Make time to talk and connect; slow down! Lubricants that are water-based (not petroleum-based) will help. Sometimes estrogen-based creams or suppositories or rings or pellets can be prescribed. My first choice is a compounded estriol suppository, but even that can cause discomfort if there is underlying inflammation or irritation. Acupuncture, craniosacral therapies and energy therapies can also help with the discomfort—as can pelvic floor physical therapy by a therapist who specializes in the pelvic floor diagnosis and treatment.

Decreased libido can also be caused by mental and emotional changes. Certainly depression can affect libido. Depression affects 10 to 20 percent of the population and is more likely to affect women then men. Most medications used to treat depression can cause a lowering of libido. Lack of sleep or increased work stress can cause changes in libido. Situational stresses such as those seen with aging parents, sick children, medical illnesses or diagnoses, financial difficulties can all interrupt our sexual lives. If there have been infidelity or trust issues in the relationship, then libido can often be affected.

Since menopause can be associated with hot flashes and sleep interruptions, we're back to the discussion of hot flashes that we had in the last section. As you can imagine, if you're not sleeping well, you're likely to be more irritable and less interested in physical intimacy. Similarly, a poor diet resulting in malnutrition or obesity can cause libido problems. Some medications such as antidepressants, beta-blockers and birth control pills can also affect libido.

Because the reasons for one person's libido change are going to be multilayered and complex, the solution is going to be individualized and similarly complicated. A nutritious and balanced diet, moderate exercise, appropriate life pacing and regular spiritual connection are essential. Focus on three or four "positives" of your partner each day. Remember what attracted you to him or her initially. Although our society might say otherwise, the organ primarily responsible for our sexual life is our brain. A frank discussion with your partner is important. Learning to communicate safely and clearly takes courage, love and patience. Professional therapists can help tremendously. Improved intimacy should be the ultimate goal. What that intimacy looks like in terms of activity and frequency of sexual activity should be decided between the two of you.

Most people equate sexual "success" with spontaneous and frequent pain-free vaginal penetration. (And certainly male medications that treat erectile dysfunction imply this is the goal of any sexual relationship!) I suggest that continuous communication is the answer.

Menopause with Hormones

What is it about the term *hormone replacement*? The very words suggest that something is "low or absent" and needs to be "replaced."

No doubt about it, the biggest issue that ob-gyn physicians face with their clients right now is the "hormone decision." We've seen a lot of column inches dedicated to understanding this controversy in newspapers, magazines and professional journals, and on the best-seller list; yet the hormone issue confuses women and some doctors. Teasing out the science and the truth from the morass of opinions takes patience and determination. The *huge* influence of big pharmaceutical companies speaking through leaders in the ob-gyn community or speaking through large marketing dollars makes it difficult to call into question any aspect of our standard of care even when there are stacks of research articles to question it!

Hormone therapy in menopause became commonly prescribed after a book by Robert Wilson called *Feminine Forever* was published (1968). Dr. Wilson proposed that estrogen would keep women feeling and looking younger and more vital. It was during this time frame that hysterectomy rates peaked in our country, and many women had their ovaries removed surgically—sometimes well before menopause. Supporting these women with patentable estrogen-like drugs was proven to help prevent osteoporosis (thinning of the bones) and atherosclerosis (hardening of the arteries). As a medical community, it became the standard of care to offer hormone "replacement" therapy to every perimenopausal and menopausal woman—even if they still had their uterus.

Now fast-forward twenty to thirty years and recognize that hysterectomy rates are lower—partly because of improved technology for surveillance (ultrasounds, MRI scans of the pelvis, smaller sampling instruments to biopsy tissue from inside the uterus) and partly because of improved technology for therapies (endometrial ablations that remove or burn the lining of the uterus and improved surgical techniques that allow smaller incisions for same-day procedures like laparoscopy or hysteroscopy).

When estrogen alone was shown to cause uterine cancer in a small percentage of women, a synthetic progestin was added and shown to "protect" the uterus. More women were on hormones than ever before. New pharmaceutical products were hitting the market one after another, and pharmaceutical companies were watching us aging baby boomers with joyful anticipation of their healthy bottom lines.

The next chapter of the hormone story begins with the first publication of the results of the Women's Health Initiative (WHI) in the summer of 2002. This study has produced lots of data and papers. Over ten thousand women were randomized to receive either placebo or Prempro (a combination of Premarin—a mix of hormones synthesized from the urine of pregnant horses—and medroxy progesterone actetate—a synthetic progestin) if they had a uterus or placebo or Premarin alone if they didn't. Although death rates were no different between the groups, there was a statistically decreased rate of colon cancer and osteoporosis and an increased rate of breast cancer, blood clots and strokes in the hormone-using groups.

The study was stopped early because the researchers believed that the risks of Prempro use outweighed the benefits. There is still an ongoing analysis of the data as we try to understand the issue. It seems that rather than answering questions, we're left with more questions to answer! What if different hormone preparations had been used? What if rather than a broad-based population we had targeted younger symptomatic women (the average age of WHI participants was sixty—well after the onset of menopause). What if we screened the population and only treated nonsmokers?

I'm amazed that there were no extensive data gathered on nutrition, life-pacing or stress management as part of the WHI. What's more, as in most clinical trials that involve taking chemicals *into* our body, there was no discussion or measurement of our individual differences in metabolizing the same chemicals *out of* our body. Our genetic uniquenesses are likely to drive this discussion in ten to fifteen years; for now we are all lumped together as if we were identical metabolically. It's unlikely that we'll ever have this large a study population to explore these questions.

In conclusion, it's clear to me that broad-based population studies give us only initial answers about risks. I'm curious about the reasons for the differences in risk among the women. It has become clear that we each have unique genetic abilities to bind hormones and to break them down and excrete them. Some of us respond to stresses better than others. Some of us eat more green vegetables. Some of us exercise more. These lifestyle choices and genetic uniquenesses are the key to approaching hormones and their "replacement."

After the WHI results were published, the pharmaceutical marketing came almost to a screeching halt. After much discussion and debate, the current standard of care is to prescribe the lowest dose of hormones needed for the shortest period of time. The North American Menopause Society has stated that all FDA-approved pharmaceutical hormones should be viewed as having the same risks and benefits.

The Bioidentical Hormone Controversy

In the last section we discussed the Women's Health Initiative, a research study sponsored by the National Institutes of Health and Wyeth Pharmaceuticals, which was designed to compare the risks and benefits of hormones in menopausal women. Since the study was funded in part by Wyeth pharmaceuticals, the choice of their drugs Premarin and Prempro was expected. As I said in the last section, over ten thousand women were randomized to receive either Prempro (a combination of Premarin—a mix of hormones synthesized from the urine of pregnant horses—and medroxy progesterone actetate—a synthetic progestin) if they had a uterus or Premarin alone if they didn't. These hormone-using women were compared to others who received a placebo drug.

Although death rates were no different between the groups, there was a lower rate of colon cancer and osteoporosis and an increased rate of breast cancer, blood clots and strokes in the hormone-using group. The study was stopped early because the researchers believed that the risk of Prempro use was greater than its benefit.

Some critics of the study point out that a different choice of hormones may have produced different results. Regardless of the source of the hormones, all of the menopausal hormone drugs produce their effect by coming into our body and attaching to hormone receptors on our cells. This connection starts a "chain reaction" of protein synthesis and metabolism. The closer the "fit" of the hormone with our cell's receptors, the closer the response is to our own hormonal responses.

When the hormones are the same as the chemicals that our bodies produce, they are termed *bioidentical.* Don't confuse this term with marketing hype such as "natural" or "derived from nature." Premarin, for example, is certainly derived from nature and is quite natural. Along the same lines, a claim that a hormone is "from plants" is another marketing term. Don't get me wrong, there are many beneficial drugs and compounds from plants (for example, aspirin from the bark of the white willow tree or digitalis from fox glove, to name just two popularly used drugs), but plant physiology is not the same as human physiology. What we find in medicine and pharmaceuticals is that the biological effectiveness of a drug is only part of the story. How the drug works in our body, how it interacts with other molecules or tissues and how our body breaks it down and excretes it safely is equally as important.

Bioidentical hormones are available in pharmaceutical and compounded formulations. The pharmaceutical hormones are FDA approved and often available on insurance formularies. There are bioidentical skin patches, topical gels, vaginal creams, vaginal rings and oral pills.

The compounded formulations are individually prescribed and prepared by specially trained pharmacists. (These formulations are not FDA approved; however, they are made from the same basic ingredients as the pharmaceutical bioidentical hormones.) The compounded drugs can also be topical, vaginal or oral preparations.

I have a preference for topical formulations—either patches, gels or creams because most women tolerate them well and their dosing is easily adjusted. Another advantage of topical delivery of the hormones is a lower risk of an elevated C-reactive protein. C-reactive protein is a nonspecific marker for inflammation. The fact that it rises slightly with oral dosing of hormones (and not with topical delivery of hormones) implies to me that oral delivery of hormonal medications sets up at least some type of inflammatory reaction as the hormone is metabolized in the liver and distributed to the body.

The hormones used can include progesterone, estradiol, estrone, estriol, testosterone and DHEA (dihydroepiandrosterone). I have chosen not to review these individually (with the exception of the discussion of estriol in the next section) and ask that you discuss their use and dosing with your gynecologist.

The biggest controversy around bioidentical hormones came recently from former actress and entrepreneur Suzanne Somers. She published two books in 2005 and 2006 (*The Sexy Years* and *The Naked Truth*), which suggested that bioidentical hormones, given in the doses and in the patterns of our reproductive years (our twenties and thirties) was the key to libido, longevity and cancer prevention. Moreover, she blasted traditional physicians for their approach to menopausal women. Needless to say, this was *not* constructive criticism that was taken to heart! Physicians and pharmaceutical companies dug in their heels and fought back with position statements and dismissive answers to their patients who were asking questions.

So what's the answer for you? As I've mentioned before, not every woman needs hormone therapy during the perimenopause or menopausal years. If you're noticing symptoms of hot flashes or changes in your sleep patterns, first explore relaxation techniques and paced breathing. We've started a biofeedback program that teaches paced breathing and shows skin temperature and pulse readouts so you can measure relaxation. Alternatively, you could set aside some time every day for relaxation, meditation or prayer.

Pay attention to your nutrition and exercise patterns. Junk food and "couch-sitting" are a bad combination. Use alcohol in moderation and don't smoke cigarettes. Consider acupuncture treatments to help the symptoms—a course of four to six treatments in combination with other lifestyle changes is usually quite effective.

If you choose to use hormones, I suggest you assess hormone levels with either serum (blood) or urine screens prior to starting them. Salivary testing can be used, but I have found it less reproducible and less reliable for female hormonal testing. My motto is "Start low, go slow"—start with a low dose of hormones for a few weeks and then adjust up if needed.

In addition to testing hormone levels, I strongly suggest you know how you personally metabolize or break down estrogen. We know that estradiol, our most biologically active female estrogen, is metabolized in our liver into several chemicals including 2-hydroxy estrone, 16α-hydroxy estrone and 4-hydroxy estrone. These chemicals can be measured in urine or blood tests through specialty laboratories. After this first phase of metabolism, the second phase then safely removes the precursors by methylation or adding a methyl group. The prevalence of each breakdown product is determined by our genetic predisposition and also our nutrition and other lifestyle habits. Once we know how we metabolize estrogen, we can modify the percentage of breakdown products with antioxidants, cruciferous vegetables, omega-3 fats and an increased dose of B vitamins and magnesium. What you need individually may be vastly different from someone else. Again, it is the combination of your genetic predisposition with your nutrition and lifestyle choices that determines the balance of estrogen breakdown products or metabolites.

Keep the lines of communication open with your physician or practitioner. I believe that the caregivers in your community want their patients to thrive during menopause. Give them the benefit of the doubt and listen. Hold their advice in your heart and decide if it's right for you.

Estriol, Wyeth Pharmaceuticals and the FDA

Let's talk about estriol. Estriol is one of the three estrogen hormones that we produce throughout our life. Even in utero there is estriol production by the growing fetus. The level is measured during pregnancy as one of the components of the triple or quad screen, a noninvasive screen for chromosomal abnormalities in the second trimester. Estriol has also been used for post-menopausal symptoms for years. It is available in Europe in several formulations and was approved by the FDA in a formulation called Hormonin here in the United States in the 1970s.

Research on estriol has been steady and continuous. There are over three hundred references on PubMed over the last thirty years on the therapeutic use of estriol without any evidence of adverse effects. Researchers at both the Medical College of Georgia in Augusta and the University of Nebraska Medical Center in Omaha have shown that estriol can have anticancer effects.

A relatively new area of research for estriol is in exploring the immune system and anti-inflammatory benefits from estriol. For instance, it may also prove to make a difference in relapsing, remitting multiple sclerosis (MS). There is currently a large multicentered trial evaluating estriol as a treatment for MS based at UCLA and funded by the National MS Society as well as the National Institutes of Health. We've known for a while, for example, that women with arthritis or psoriasis or other autoimmune conditions usually have fewer symptoms during their pregnancies when serum estriol levels are high.

I've used estriol in my patients for almost twenty years. It is especially helpful for atrophic vaginitis (post-menopausal thinning of the vagina) and in combination with estradiol for recalcitrant menopausal symptoms such as hot flashes or night sweats.

And now our story grows a little stranger. On October 6, 2005, Wyeth Pharmaceuticals, the maker of Premarin and Prempro, filed a "citizen's petition" with the Food and Drug Administration (FDA) stating that estriol should not be used because it was not FDA approved and that compounded hormones that contained estriol "pose a serious threat to public health." The irony of this statement (other than the fact that a naturally occurring hormone was being singled out by this pharmaceutical company) is that Wyeth currently has a European drug on the market that contains estriol.

To my dismay, many professional organizations such as the North American Menopause Society (NAMS) and the American College of Obstetricians and Gynecologists (ACOG) stepped up to agree with Wyeth. I note with interest that, without exception, every organization that agreed with the statement receives money in some way from the company. Half of the board members of NAMS have received consulting fees from Wyeth. Wyeth endows a lectureship in the name of the past president of NAMS, Dr. Wulf Utian. And the list goes on. I'll spare you the depressing details—they are a matter of public record, but believe me when I tell you that money moves strongly through my profession's peer-reviewed journals and "Committee Opinions."

On the other hand, many clinicians and citizens filed comments in support of estriol use with the FDA in response to Wyeth's complaint. As a matter of fact, the FDA received over 77,000 comments—a record response. Despite strong public sentiment, the FDA responded in January 2008 by sending letters warning seven pharmacies to stop using estriol. The pharmacies were also warned to stop claiming that their compounded hormones were better than other hormones available.

You may be surprised to learn that I agree with this part of the statement—although there are data to support the use of natural progesterone over synthetic progestins such as medroxy-progesterone acetate (Provera), I believe it is inappropriate to claim superior safety with compounded hormones. The only way to improve safety of hormone use is to ensure that the body safely metabolizes the hormones that are taken in—and that has everything to do with genetic predisposition and nutrition. I am also a strong advocate of regular mammography and the exploration on nonhormonal treatments for menopausal symptoms such as acupuncture and biofeedback therapy whenever possible.

Clinicians were told that they could use estriol if they filed an Investigational New Drug (IND) application. (So far, at least, the FDA did not chastise pregnant mothers for making estriol naturally!)

The end of this chapter on estriol is still being written. Congress has stepped in, and House resolution HR342 demanded the FDA reverse its plan to stop prescription compounding with estriol; the Senate passed a resolution S5456 with similar verbiage. If nothing else, Wyeth has managed to mobilize a large cadre of pharmacists, clinicians and patients who are educating themselves and speaking their minds. Ah, democracy! I have to believe the truth will eventually come out about estriol; perhaps a new presidency and a less industry-tied FDA will make the difference. Unfortunately I am less optimistic about the professional societies that represent the medical profession—but I'm ready to be pleasantly surprised!

7

Grace and Balance in the Cycle of Life—a Postscript

There is a vitality, a life force, an energy, a quickening that is translated through you into action, and because there is only one of you in all time, this expression is unique. And if you block it, it will never exist through any other medium and will be lost.

Martha Graham

Life-force energy is the drive to grow and flourish despite rocky or challenging conditions. It is the grass pushing up between the cracks in asphalt or concrete. It is the ability to push through illness toward optimal health and balance. It is the continuing ability to tap into our body's innate drive to heal. Grace, by definition, is unmerited divine assistance for regeneration or sanctification. Grace is the "fuel" for our life-force energy. We need our divine connection to remember our physical health that has been fragmented because of our lifestyle choices or life circumstances. We need grace to replenish our emotional health. We need grace to reconnect to our spiritual source.

Many of us have had times in our life when the drive to heal has been blunted by excesses. Perhaps the excesses were in alcohol or recreational drug use. Perhaps the excesses were in pushing ourselves at work or at school until that project was completed or that term paper was written. Regardless of the source, it is possible to blunt or attenuate our life force energy. But even after excesses and overuse there is still a spark that is ready to be fanned into flame.

After every inspiration, there is an expiration. After a drive to achieve, there is a need for rest. After the magic of creation, there was a day of rest. I leave you with the inner knowledge that imbalance or disease is a cue to reread the chapter on lifestyle and nutrition. Reconnect to your inner wisdom and find that emotional, physical and spiritual balance that brings you to optimal health.

Be well!

References

Introduction

The Institute for Functional Medicine, PO Box 1697, Gig Harbor, WA 98335, www.functionalmedicine.org.

Life Success Seminars, PO Box 1369, West Chester, OH 45071, (513) 874-0555, www.lifesuccessseminars.com.

Natural Rhythms, Lisa Michaels, PO Box 3654, Lilburn, GA 30048, www.naturalrhythms.org.

Warren, M.P. 2008. Low dose HRT options. *Menopause Management*, Nov/Dec: 28–29.

Lifestyle

Bennett, G.G. et al. 2006. Television viewing and pedometer-determined physical activity among multiethnic residents of low-income housing. *Am J Pub Health* 96:1681–85.

Bertone-Johnson, E.R. et al. 2005. Calcium and vitamin D intake and risk of incident premenstrual syndrome. *Arch Int Med* 165(11):1246–52.

Blot, W.J. et al. 1993. Nutrition intervention trials in Linxian, China. *J. Natl Cancer Inst* 85:1483–91.

Bodnar, L. 2007. Vitamin D deficiency widespread during pregnancy. *ScienceDaily* 10 March, http://www.sciencedaily. com/releases/2007/02/070227105140.htm.

Cummings, D.E. and D.R. Flum. 2008. Gastrointestinal surgery as a treatment for diabetes. *JAMA* 299(3): 341–43.

ConsumerLab. Private lab that does testing of over-the-counter supplements, www.consumerlab.com.

Dixon, J.B., P.E. O'Brien PE, et al. 2008. Adjustable gastric banding and conventional therapy for type 2 diabetes: A randomized controlled trial. *JAMA* 299(3):316–23.

Halvorsen, B.L. et al. 2002. A systematic screening of total antioxidants in dietary plants. *J. Nutr* 132:461–71.

Kimball, S.M. et al. 2007. Safety of vitamin D3 in adults with multiple sclerosis. *Am J Clin Nutr* 86(3):645–51.

Lemley, B. 2004. What does science say you should eat?

Discover Magazine 5 Feb. http://discovermagazine.com/2004/feb/science-diet.

Liva, Rick. 2007. *Integrative Medicine* Oct/Nov 2007.

Oldways. Web site reviews different food pyramids for different cultures, www.oldwayspt.org.

Pellegrini, N. et al. 2003. Total antioxidant capacity of plant foods, beverages and oils consumed in Italy assessed by three different in vitro assays. *J Nutr* 133: 2812–19.

Prochaska, J. et al. 1994. *Changing for Good:A Revolutionary Six-Stage Program for Overcoming Bad Habits and Moving Your Life Positively Forward.* Avon Books.

Rogan, E.G. et al. 2003. Relative imbalances in estrogen metabolism and conjugation in breast tissue of women with carcinoma: Potential biomarkers of susceptibility to cancer. *Carcinogenesis* 22(9):697–702.

Smith, Bob L. 1993. Organic foods vs. supermarket foods: Element levels. *Journal of Applied Nutrition* 45(1):35–39.

Steingrimsdottir, L. et al. 2005. Relationship between serum parathyroid hormone levels, vitamin D sufficiency, and calcium intake. *JAMA* 294:2336–41.

Suzuki, A. et al. 2006. Hypovitaminosis D in type 2 diabetes mellitus: Association with microvascular complications and type of treatment. *Endocr J* 53(4):503–10.

Swithers, S.E. and T.L. Davidson. 2008. A role for sweet taste: Calorie predictive relations in energy regulation by rats. *Behavioral Neuroscience* 122 (1):161–73.

Warburton, D.E.R. et al. 2006. Health benefits of physical activity: The evidence. *CMAJ* 174(6):801–9.

You, W.C. et al. 2005. Etiology and prevention of gastric cancer: A population study in a high risk area of China. *Chinese J Dig Dis* 6(4):149–54.

The Integrative Medicine Toolbox

Acupuncture

Helms, J. 2007. *Acupuncture Energetics: A Clinical Approach for Physicians*. Medical Acupuncture Publishers.

Helms, J. 2007. *Getting to Know You*. Random House.

Guided Imagery

Blankfield, R.P. 1991. Suggestion, relaxation, and hypnosis as adjuncts in the care of surgery patients: A review of the literature. *Am J Clin Hypn* 33(3):172–86.

Kaushik, R. et al. 2005. Biofeedback assisted diaphragmatic breathing and systematic relaxation versus propranolol in long term prophylaxis of migraine. *Complement Ther Med* 13(3):165–74.

Nunes, D.F.T. et al. 2007. Relaxation and guided imagery program in patients with breast cancer undergoing radiotherapy is not associated with neuroimmunomodulatory effects. *J Psychosom Res* 63(6):647–55.

Paul-Labrador, M. et al. 2006. Effects of a randomized controlled trial of transcendental meditation on components of the metabolic syndrome in subjects with coronary heart disease. *Arch Int Med* 166(11):1218–24.

Understanding the Cycle of Life

Northrup, C. 2006. *Women's Bodies Women's Wisdom.* HayHouse.

Fibroids

Mehl-Madrona, L. 2002. Complementary medicine treatment of uterine fibroids: A pilot study. *Alt Ther* 8(2):34–46.

Chiaffarino, F. et al. 1999. Diet and uterine myomas. *Obstets Gynecol* 94:395–98.

Menopause

Kuehn, B.M. 2008. FDA warns claims for pharmacy-made "bio-identical" hormones are misleading. *JAMA* 299:512.

Wilson, R. 1968. *Feminine Forever.* Pocket Books.

About the Author

Dr. Claudia Harsh is a board-certified obstetrician/gynecologist who has been the Director of Integrative Gynecology at the Alliance Institute for Integrative Medicine in Cincinnati, Ohio since September 2003. The Bravewell Collaborative chose the Alliance Institute as one of eight national centers for excellence in clinical integrative medicine in 2004. Prior to joining the Alliance Institute, Dr. Harsh was the co-founder of Crescent Women's Medical Group in Cincinnati and practiced general obstetrics and gynecology for 14 years. Dr. Harsh is currently enrolled in the University of Arizona's two-year Fellowship in Integrative Medicine that was begun by Andrew Weil, M.D.

Dr. Harsh has written monthly columns for *Cincinnati Women's Magazine* on integrative gynecology since 2007 and is a sought-after speaker on a wide variety of women's health and wellness topics.

Index